MINDFUL EATING

Thirty Days to A Whole New You

KAREN MAYO

ISBN: 150234856X
ISBN 13: 9781502348562
Library of Congress Control Number: 2014916499
CreateSpace Independent Publishing Platform
North Charleston, South Carolina

GRATITUDE

I am grateful for the Lord, who is blessing me with abundance every day in every way.

I am grateful for my mom and my dad who always encouraged me to keep moving forward and to follow my dreams.

I am grateful for my grandmother who inspired me in so many ways.

I am grateful for the people in my life who have continued to inspire me, mentor me, coach me, and support me here on this earth, and I am grateful for the people who have positively influenced me who are no longer with us. I'm so grateful to have been blessed with your presence.

I am grateful for my nephew, Scott. He is the reason I decided to enroll in the Institute for Integrative Nutrition.

I am grateful for Joshua Rosenthal, principal of the Institute for Integrative Nutrition, for having a vision of the ripple effect.

Cheers to you. I'm hoping you find something that can lead to a positive change in your health and well-being.

It is an easy positive affirmation to say aloud things you are grateful for every day, or you can even tell someone that you are grateful for that person, and then explain why.

"Let food be thy medicine
and medicine be thy food"
–Hippocrates

TABLE OF CONTENTS

Introduction

xi

My Intention

xvi

"Why I Do What I Do"

xix

and My Motivation

xxiii

Chapter One

Chronic Conditions

1

Food and Mood Connection

4

Seasonal Eating and The Benefits

6

Spices, Herbs, and Teas and Their Health Benefits

10

Superfoods or Just Plain Food?

13

To Go Organic or Not? That is the Question

26

What Does Mindful Eating Mean?

34

"A Rainbow of Foods"

38

Chapter Two

Have you Checked Your pH Today?

41

Nine reasons why you need to have a balanced pH

42

Chapter Three

Do You Have the Sugar Blues?

50

The Aging Connection

51

The good, bad, and Basic Material of Life

54

What causes Cravings?

60

Chapter Four

The Raw Differences

63

Why are we so sick?

63

Juicing Has no Pulp

64

Smoothies Have Pulp

66

Cleansing and Detoxing and Fasting Oh My!

69

Chapter Five
Prepare for the Mindful Eating Menu Plan
78
Phase One-Prepare to Cleanse Your Bloodstream
79
Phase Two-The Transition
83
Phase Three-An Optional Phase
85

Chapter Six
The Mindful-Eating Meal Program
86
Tips for Eating Out
88
Week One and Two
90—112
Week Three and Four
113—140
Week Five-Optional
141
Recipes
142
Handbook
144
Symptom List
144
Mindful, Daily Helpful Tips
147
Good Food Choice List
150
Weekly Shopping List
154
Daily Mindful Eating Program
156

$\mathcal{I}$ NTRODUCTION

$\mathcal{W}$ e all know, or have known, someone who is sick with a chronic illness: a grandparent, parent, sister, brother, aunt, uncle, cousin, spouse, or friend. These illnesses are prevalent and run through generations.

How did this happen to us?

The way our grandparents, and even our parents, ate is much different from how we are eating today. The increased population and mechanization of the United States economy has led us away from farm fresh, natural foods and toward commercialized and processed foods.

Our ancestors ate from the land, either food from a local farm or from their own garden. Their diets consisted of fresh and organic produce. Farmers maintained quality soil that had essential nutrients and minerals by mulching, rotating crops, and adding manure. That soil produced quality plants, which in turn nourished the animals that fed on those plants.

After World War II, everything changed. Companies that once made weapons were now making chemicals for fertilizers. They promised the farmers a way to increase the growth of their crops and animals, while decreasing annoying insects. Today, U.S. farmers use about three billion pounds of chemical pesticides on their crops. Authorities estimate that 45 percent of the vegetables that are offered for sale contain traces of pesticides. Chemical fertilizers also strip the soil of essential nutrients such as calcium for healthy bones, magnesium for energy and muscle function, and selenium for strong hearts. If these nutrients are not present in the soil, they are certainly not in the food we buy. Mineral content levels in our commercial foods have fallen by more than 40 percent in the last fifty years.

We also need to look at food processing, how food gets transported, and where we buy our food. Food processing strips away nutrients and commercialized processed meats reduce levels of vitamin B6, which is essential for the immune system and brain function. Freezing can destroy B1 and B2 vitamins, which are needed for energy. Also, the longer it takes food to reach our stores and our tables, both vitamins A and C are degraded.

Portion sizes have changed in the past fifty years too. It's called "portion distortion." A brownie recipe from the *Joy of Cooking* cookbook, printed in the 1960s, makes a much smaller brownie than the recipes of today. How much smaller? Half as big. Since recipes are written to make more, people have the option to eat more...and they are eating more.

Rates of obesity and heart attacks are a major public-health problem in the United States, and these rates continue to increase. Poor diet is linked to heart disease, diabetes, stroke, arthritis, respiratory disease, oral conditions, and certain cancers.

Food-related disease is the number-one cause of preventable death in the United States. Other health conditions such as ADD, IBS, gout, asthma, and allergies are rapidly increasing around the world as other countries adopt Western eating habits.

As a result more people than ever are on prescription medication for chronic illness. Insurance premiums are the highest in history. Medication costs are on the rise, and doctors spend less and less time with their patients.

The answer to the twenty-first century health crisis is not increasing medications or having an operation. The solution to getting our health on track starts with simply getting back into the kitchen and going back to the basics. Eating healthy and living a healthy lifestyle is the answer.

You might be surprised at the small changes that can make a big difference. The recommendations you will discover in this book are easy, and we can work toward a healthy lifestyle together.

Just remember that a healthy lifestyle is a lifetime transition of healthy eating.

—Karen Mayo

NOTE TO READERS

This publication contains the opinion, experience, and ideas of its author. It is intended to provide helpful and informative material on the subjects addressed. It is not the intention of the author and publisher to render any medical, health, psychological, or any other kind of personal or professional services. The reader should consult his or her medical or health professional before adopting any of the suggestions in this book.

The author and the publisher specifically disclaim all responsibility for any liability, loss, or risk, personal or otherwise, which is incurred as a consequence, directly or indirectly, of the use and application of any of the contents of this book.

DISCLAIMER

The dietary suggestions and recipes contained in this book are not intended to replace the service of a trained health professional. All matters regarding your health require medical supervision. You should consult your physician before adopting the suggestions of this book. Any applications of the treatments set forth in this book are at the reader's discretion.

My intention for this book is to share with you what I've learned about healing our bodies with food.

I wish I had known about this healing before I lost my mom to cancer and my grandparents to chronic diseases. I want to share with you how easy it is to make healthier choices in what you are eating and to help yourself back to living a healthy lifestyle.

How is this book different? I certainly don't have all the answers. But this is my perspective on what I have learned through research and lived through experiences of my own life. I will be sharing with you a few things we never learned in health class. I hope you truly learn something new and that you experience a few aha moments.

I know this way of eating works because my clients are losing weight, thinking more clearly, feeling more energetic, and best of all they are able to come off their medications.

There comes a time in ones life as it has in mine that you want to make a difference for humanity this is my small contribution to that pledge. A driving dream in my life was to create a piece of my passion to help humanity. This book is a small piece of the delivery of that promise. We all make promises every day to ourselves, to our families, to our colleagues and to our communities. You the reader matter to me, this book is not only about wellness, nutrition and health. It is about what matters, you matter. As a young girl growing up on a farm in Pennslyvania I learned about eating; in this book I hope you will learn as I have about living. Growing up in Pennslyvania with my mom, dad and two sisters. A hard working American family, living the American dream during the 70's. We had pigs, cows and a big half acre size garden, which had everything from green beans, tomatoes, broccoli, cucumbers to lettuces and peppers. My sister, Dawn and I used to pick weeds on the weekends and feed them to the cows and pigs, not our favorite thing to do as teenagers but looking back on it now, how I was raised was a great way to grow up. My mother's cooking was the best and I learned a lot from her. I have had a widely varied careers working as a bartender, sous chef, model, actress, licensed real estate agent, home mortgage banker, motivational speaker and executive recruiter. Along the way I always kept my family roots to a healthy way of eating. My passion is teaching others how making small changes in eating healthy can make a big difference in healing their bodies and also in gut health. I am a board certified holistic nutrition health and lifestyle coach. As a health coach, I am your personal advocate for living; I am board certified member of American Association of Drugless Practitioners. I am certified as a healthy eating specialist. I am co-founder of Mahopac Health Coaching, located inside of Bad Mikey's in Mahopac, New York; I work with groups and one on one coaching at my office. I also partner with corporations to present wellness workshops. I have most recently become a bee-keeper. All the integrated pieces of us as a work of art coming together in healthy living to continue to be vibrant to all that matters to us. As you judge this book for its value know that I believe in your value.

Chapter one shares a bit about what I think is important for the reader to understand in order to get the most out of this book. I write about mindful eating, chronic illness conditions, whole foods, seasonal eating, and much more.

Chapter two you may learn about a new concept. Have you ever heard of checking the pH levels in your body? No? I hadn't for most of my adult life either.

I learned that the food we eat creates either an acidic or alkaline environment in our body, which then affects our blood level. How? If our body is too acidic, that creates trouble, and if it's too alkaline, that also creates trouble. So we need to be in the middle. In chapter two I will share with you what I have learned in this fascinating area, including the supporting research.

Chapter three is about sugar and how it relates to aging. You will learn about the glycemic index and how sugar ties in with chronic illness.

Chapter four is about juicing, smoothies, and the differences between a detox, a cleanse, and fasting.

Chapter five is a five-week meal plan with recipes. This chapter is a step-by-step program with a life-changing menu. I know it works because I am already seeing results with my clients. Many are off their medications completely, or they have had the medication dosage lowered. You can do this step-by-step program at any time of the year, ideally at the change of each season. This program allows for a slow transition, which makes for a healthier and happier lifestyle. Each time you go through the program, you will switch to healthier eating habits.

Chapter six is a workbook with a shopping list, and a personal food and nutrition journal.

"WHY I DO WHAT I DO"

My nephew, Scott, came to stay with me during his sixth-grade school year, which was fall of 2011 through spring of 2012. His mother, my sister, is a single mom who has been enlisted in the United States Army. She wanted to make a difference in her son's life. Scott was not able to go to South Carolina to boot camp with her, so she asked if he could stay with me. "Of course," I said. Prior to Scott coming to live with me, he was eating everything from fast food to frozen TV dinners that he cooked himself. Doritos were his favorite snack. He was on ADHD medication, and his grades were a C at best. Scott was eating unhealthy foods loaded with chemicals and preservatives. No wonder he was not thinking at his best, which his grades clearly demonstrated.

We established a new routine. We ate breakfast in the morning. I would pack his lunch almost every day, and then we would eat a healthy dinner. One of his teachers called me and said she and the other teachers would like to set up a meeting with me. I had no idea why. I thought maybe Scott needed his medication. Scott never came to my house with his medication for ADHD, I was not having that medication in my house when it did not seem like he needed it from my perspective. I went to the meeting, and something magical happened. I sat at a table and listened to Scott's teachers tell me how pleased they are with him. Off of his medications and eating healthy, Scott had earned a place on the honor roll and received a certificate from the Blue Mountain Middle School for straight As in math. His math teacher told me that she was in awe of him when she would watch him multiply three numbers by three numbers and arrive at the correct answer without using scratch paper. I couldn't say anything. I just stared at his teachers in shock. "What are you doing with him?" they asked. The teachers were finding it hard to understand how Scott could have such a big turnaround when they looked at his past records. I said I was just doing what my mother did with my sisters and me. I was feeding him healthy, nutritious food. Scott was eating much healthier, so his brain and body were healthy.

Scott also bloomed in other areas. He played baseball on a Little League team and received his first trophy, and he was also an active Boy Scout.

I thought, *If I can do this with a sixth grader, then I need to get out and talk to people about how easy it is to eat healthy and get off their medications. That small change can make a big difference.*

My journey led me to Institute for Integrative Nutrition, which is the world's largest nutrition school per graduating class. Powerful teachers who are the leading doctors, PhDs, researchers, and authorities in nutrition today taught me a wide variety of skills in business, coaching, nutrition, and lifestyle choices.

I graduated in June 2013, board certified by Institute of Intregrative Nutrition as a Holistic Health Practitioner, certified by the American Association of Drugless Practitioners and a member of International Association of Health Coaches. Certified Corporate Wellness Presenter. I now offer programs to clients ranging from a thirty-day kick-start program to a lifestyle change consultation, which can be for as long as you need me. I also offer my clients one-on-one coaching, as well as group coaching with wellness workshops, lunch and learns, wellness presentations to corporations, cooking classes, grocery store tours, health-food store tours, and so much more.

My Motivation

I know there are people who are sick from their chronic illness and can't sleep at night because of something they ate or their medications. My motivation is to meet those people and to be of service to them so they can heal their bodies. If you know someone who can use this book, please pass it on. Once you know the fundamentals in this book, you will know how to learn, live, and love a healthy lifestyle.

As I would say, "No more (die)ting it's about living!"

CHAPTER ONE

CHRONIC CONDITIONS

*I*n the United States, we have a public health crisis called chronic-disease conditions.

A chronic condition is a health condition or disease that is persistent or otherwise long lasting in its effects or a disease that comes with time. The term "chronic" is usually applied when the course of the disease lasts for more than three months.

Obesity and heart attacks are major public health problems in the United States, and they continue to increase. These chronic conditions are not just at home where you live; the ramifications of these chronic conditions also follow you to your workplace.

The main health concerns we face center around eight health risks and behaviors, including poor diet, alcohol consumption, sleep deprivation, physical inactivity, poor self-care, poor stress management, smoking, and lack of health screening. These risks drive and impact the fifteen most common chronic conditions, which in turn account for 80 percent of the total cost for all chronic conditions. Chronic disease conditions cause about 70 percent of all deaths each year in the United States. The impact of these fifteen conditions on an employer's medical spending typically exceeds 65 percent of the bottom line. Employers who can target and impact just three of the eight will see a significant savings per employee.

The common chronic conditions that are most often seen in the workplace are diabetes, heart disease, hypertension, back pain, obesity, cancer, asthma, arthritis, allergies, sinusitis, depression, high blood pressure, kidney disease, liver disease, and high cholesterol.

By reducing the frequency and severity of the most costly chronic medical conditions, employers can begin to gain control of healthcare costs, improve health and performance of their employees, and build their business for better health.

While risk factors vary with age and gender, most of the common chronic diseases are caused by the food people eat, their lifestyle choices, and metabolic risk factors. These factors are also responsible for the resulting mortality rates. Therefore, these conditions might be prevented by behavioral changes, such as quitting smoking, adopting a healthy diet, and increasing physical activity. Social determinants are important risk factors for chronic diseases. Social factors such as financial stability, education level, and ethnicity, are also a major factor of chronic disease. The hurdles in medical care can complicate patient monitoring and their motivation to continue to go to treatment. In addition to these factors, overuse of antibiotics has recently been associated with chronic liver disease.

When you improve eating habits, you will experience sustained energy and reduced stress, And when you increase healthy lifestyle activities, like self-care and exercise, you will feel improved overall health, reduced stress and anxiety, and an increase in energy and vitality.

The American Heart Association recommends healthy lifestyle habits such as exercise and fitness. Thirty minutes of physical activity will add up to a healthier heart and reduce the risk for a heart attack. Having a healthy eating plan means choosing the right foods to eat and preparing those foods in a healthy way. It can actually be easy to eat healthy, and I will share my simple plan later in the book.

Food and Mood Connection

I would like to briefly talk about the food and mood connection; what we eat or drink does affect our mood. Consider how most people feel when they drink coffee or alcohol. These two stimulants will affect your mood in less than sixty minutes. The standard American diet (SAD, for short) is high in processed carbohydrates and poor-quality processed animal protein. As mentioned previously, even the vegetables and fruits that we do eat are lacking vitamins and nutrients, and this poor SAD diet results in bad moods. It's hard to feel inspired and happy when you're living on chemicals and artificial junk food.

Here is the scientific perspective. The food-mood relationship is maintained by neurotransmitters—chemical messengers that relay thoughts and actions throughout the brain.

Neurotransmitters, such as serotonin, make us feel relaxed. An example of this is the feeling you get when you eat carbohydrates like pasta. Eating too many carbs or overly processed carbs, like sugar and flour, releases more serotonin, which causes drowsiness.

Eating protein produces a neurotransmitter, dopamine, which has a stimulating effect on the brain. It makes you feel full of energy if eaten in appropriate portions. On the other hand, overeating protein can lead to tension and irritability.

The food we eat breaks down in our digestive track then enters our bloodstream and creates changes in the behavior of these two neurotransmitters, which in turn impacts our mood.

Another example of the food-and-mood connection is how we typically feel at Thanksgiving. In order to handle the excess of food that we eat, the blood flow is directed to the stomach and away from the brain, so we then feel lethargic.

Each person's food-and-mood connection is different. Only you can determine the right amount of protein, carbohydrate, and fats to keep yourself balanced.

Keep a food-and-water journal to track what you are eating, how you are feeling within an hour after eating, and how much water you're drinking. (Drink half your body weight in ounces. So if you weigh two hundred pounds, drink one hundred ounces of water a day.)

S EASONAL E ATING AND THE B ENEFITS

$\mathcal{T}$he seasons of spring, summer, fall, and winter form the never-ending circle of life. No matter where you live, each season brings an opportunity to delight our taste buds with new fruits, vegetables, herbs, and spices. When we take advantage of locally grown, seasonal foods, we are helping our bodies to make the transition from one season to the next more easily—not to mention that fresh local foods taste much better then processed foods. Another advantage of seasonal eating is that, since the produce is grown locally, there is less risk of contamination during transportation, less fuel is used, and less waste is released in the environment.

Eating seasonally is an easy, healthy habit to create. Our ancestors ate seasonally because they had no choice. Families harvested each seasonal crop and understood the importance of canning, freezing, and proper storing.

Today, most of us don't even know which foods are in season. We go to the store and pick up whatever we want. Stores have everything from strawberries during the winter season to winter squash during the summer season. We have no clue as to when it arrived, how it got there, or where it came from. Most of us fill our carts with what looks good, cook our meals, and call it a day. The next time you reach for produce, look at the label to see if the food was grown in the United States. I will talk more about the labels, the numbers, and what they mean later in the book.

Our cooking methods are sometimes naturally seasonal. During summer we fire up the outside grill, and we tend to eat more raw foods like salads and foods that are light and cooling to our bodies. During the winter when it's cold and dry, we want foods that are moist and warm—perhaps using the crockpot. We tend to gravitate toward stews, soups, and heavy, warming foods.

Here's a look at what is most likely available by the season. Use this as a guide to healthier seasonal eating. When you are eating with the seasons, you can enjoy the rainbow of colorful and diverse whole foods, and you will be providing your body with a wide variety of important vitamins, minerals, enzymes, antioxidants, and phytochemicals that you need to create a healthy lifestyle.

Spring—During this season your health focus is on lightening up. Cooking methods are baking, sautéing, toasting, and grilling.

Foods—Artichokes, apricots, arugula, asparagus, avocados, beetroot, carrots, chicory, collards, cherries, dandelion greens, fennel, garlic, green beans, honeydew melons, kiwifruit, limes, lychees, mangoes, mustard greens, new potatoes, oranges, pineapple, raspberries, rhubarb, spinach, strawberries, spring lettuce, Swiss chard, sugar-snap and snow peas, onions, watercress

Herbs—Sage, rosemary, thyme, tarragon, parsley, chives, and basil

Summer—In the summer season, your health focus is hydration and cooling. Cooking methods are sautéing, grilling, and lightly steaming.

Food—Apricots, bell peppers, blackberries, blueberries, broccoli, cantaloupe, carrots, cherries, corn, cucumbers, eggplants, grapes, green beans, honeydew melons, lettuce, mangoes, nectarines, passion fruit, peaches, pineapple, plums, potatoes, raspberries, strawberries, sugar-snap peas, summer squash, tomatoes, watermelon, zucchini

Herbs—Basil, cayenne, cilantro, coriander, parsley, and peppermint

Fall—Now your seasonal health focus is storing energy and building up your immune system. Cooking methods are baking, steaming, stir-frying, roasting, sautéing, and braising.

Foods—Acorn squash, apples, broccoli, brussels sprouts, Swiss chard, carrots, cauliflower, cranberries, eggplants, fennel, figs, grapes, kale, lemons, olives, onions, parsnips, pears, permissions, potatoes, pome-granates, pumpkin, quince, sweet potatoes, turnips, wild mushrooms, winter squash (like butternut and spaghetti squash)

Herbs—Allspice, cloves, cinnamon, ginger, mustard seeds and peppercorns

Winter—During the winter season, your health focus is to reserve en-ergy and rest. Cooking methods are baking, slow-cooking stews and soups, lightly steaming, and roasting.

Foods—Apples, avocado, bananas, broccoli, broccoli rabe, brussels sprout, Belgian endive, cabbage, carrots, cauliflower, chestnuts, dates, fennel, ruby grapefruit, kale, leeks, lemon, lime, kiwifruit, onions, oranges, parsnips, pears, radicchio, radishes, persimmons, rutabaga, sweet potatoes, tangerines, turnips, and winter squash (like acorn, butternut, and spaghetti squash).

When you are shopping at the supermarkets, you will see fruits and vegetables that are available when they are not in season. Many of these out-of-season, nonorganic foods depend on waxes, chemicals, and preservatives to make them look fresh and to make them look perfect and appear more delicious than they actually are. These foods are produced for a longer shelf life rather than for flavor.

When you can't find fresh seasonal foods, check the freezer section of the store. Foods are picked at their best, and then they are flash frozen at that time. These foods can be a great alternative to buying foods that are out of season.

I make a conscious effort to buy seasonal foods and to support my local farmers. I feel more connected to the food on my plate, which makes me feel more grounded. Organic, seasonal foods are grown by farmers who rotate crops to increase the soil fertility, use beneficial insects instead of toxic pesticides, and use sustainable composting. Using these sustainable methods of growing food, the local farmers produce quality food with minerals, vitamins, enzymes, and phyto-chemicals that commercialized, conventional processes cannot match.

Seasonal foods offer a natural diversity that we should take advantage of when eating, as nature intended to sustain both our health and the health of the planet. Once you create the habit of eating season-ally, you will enjoy the benefits of better-tasting food and a healthier lifestyle.

SPICES, HERBS, AND TEAS AND THEIR HEALTH BENEFITS

Common herbs and spices have powerful inflammation-fighting properties and may help protect against certain chronic illnesses such as diabetes, heart disease, and some cancers. Herbs and spices can add appealing flavor to your meals, and they are also a healthier option than salt, fat, and sugar.

When purchasing dried herbs and spices, look for the "best by" dates on the packages, and store the herbs in an airtight container away from heat, moisture, and direct sunlight. If you are using fresh herbs or spices, double the amount to get the same levels of active substances that are in their dried counterparts.

Let us take a closer look at some herbs, which come from plants or plant parts.

Basil has antibacterial, antiseptic, and antifungal properties. It stimulates the immune system by increasing the production of antibodies. Basil oil can provide relief for asthma, sinus congestion, arthritis, and headaches.

Chamomile is frequently used as a relaxing tea that also aids in digestion and the production of urine.

Dandelion is an important tonic good source of potassium. It also aids the liver by, it reducing congestion and improving the flow of bile, and it supports the kidneys by enhancing the flow of urine.

Fennel acts as a digestive aid to relieve cramps. It may also stimulate appetite. This herb should be avoided during pregnancy.

Ginger has natural anti-inflammatory properties and also circulatory and digestive benefits. It eases nausea due to morning sickness, motion sickness, and chemotherapy. It's worth considering for arthritis, sore throats, and congestion.

Parsley may reduce the risk of liver cancer. Parsley is a good diuretic for helping to flush the kidneys of toxins. It is also high in antioxidants and supports and strengthens the liver.

Rosemary eases migraines and tension headaches when taken as a tea. It can also relieve exhaustion and fatigue.

Thyme is known for its ability to ease bronchial inflammation.

Now let's turn our attention to spices. Spices often come from the seeds, berries, bark, or roots of plants.

Cayenne or chili peppers get their heat from capsaicin, which is a compound that's been shown in early studies to help protect against cancer. It may help stave off hunger and boost fat-burning calories. Capsaicin also has the potential to relieve pain and the power to lower blood pressure and stimulate circulation and metabolism.

Cinnamon is an antioxidant linked to lower inflammation. It has been shown to reduce blood glucose levels in people with diabetes.

Turmeric is the most potent antioxidant spice. It is a relative to ginger. Turmeric prevents cancer, known to releve arthritis, control diabetes, and reduce cholesterol level, boosts the immune system, heals wounds faster, improves digestion and prevents liver disease.

Garlic is a potent antibacterial, antiviral, and anticancer spice. It has also been found to prevent blood clotting, lower blood pressure, and reduce inflammation.

Tea is truly a health beverage with astonishing benefits, due to the polyphenols they contain.

White tea is the least processed tea. It has a delicate flavor and is a delicious source of antioxidants as well as being low in caffeine. White tea promotes hydration and supports general health and the complexion.

Green tea should have a nutty flavor when freshly brewed. This tea has the potential to lower LDL (bad) cholesterol. Green tea helps support the immune system, and it can help maintain healthy blood-sugar levels.

Oolong tea is in-between green and black tea in flavor and antioxidant activity. Oolong comes in many varieties, from fruity to flowery, and promotes a healthy metabolism. It may also help support digestion and help promote healthy skin and teeth.

Black tea is a hearty tea that can range in flavor from nutty to spicy to fruity and flowery. This tea is energy boosting and helps to promote heart health. Black tea also helps maintain healthy cardiovascular and circulatory systems.

SUPERFOODS OR JUST PLAIN FOOD?

The term "Superfoods" refers to foods that are full of health benefits and have the highest concentration of nutrients, vitamins and antioxidants. They are powerful enough to help lower cholesterol, boost the immune system, enhance sexuality, cleanse and alkalize the body, lower inflammation, reduce the risk of heart disease and some cancer, and improve mood.

Some superfoods are rich in nutrients that are good for your skin and hair. Others are particularly high in free-radical scavenging antioxidants that may help prevent many common chronic diseases and slow down the visible signs of aging. Many superfoods are full of important vitamins, minerals, essential fatty acids, enzymes, and other beneficial compounds that can improve your health, nourish our body at the cellular level, and increase your energy and state of mental health. There are a lot of superfoods out there, and with their growing popularity and dramatic low prices, there has never been a better time to start eating superfoods.

Fruits and berries contain extremely high levels of antioxidants that prevent free-radical damage and slow visible signs of aging. When they are eaten regularly, they can have an amazing effect on your overall energy levels and well-being.

Goji berries are packed with protein and iron, and they contain every type of essential amino acids. They are also rich in vitamin A. Goji berries can be purchased dried in either whole or powdered form. You can enjoy eating them raw with chocolate, or add them to a smoothie.

Camu berries are an amazing source of vitamin C, crucial antioxidant that helps to neutralize free radicals responsible for many chronic diseases and accelerated aging. Our bodies can't make it on their own, so we have to get vitamin C from the foods we eat. Just one serving of camu camu powder contains about 1180% of your daily vitamin C value – you'd have to eat more than 10 oranges to get the same amount. Camu berries can also help your body rebuild tissue, boost immunity, and increase energy. They are also great for eye health. Camu berries can be purchased in powdered form and added to smoothies or sprinkled on desserts.

Strawberries, raspberries, and blackberries are all superfoods, but blueberries exceed them all in health benefits. Eating only four ounces of blueberries provides the same amount of age-defying antioxidants as five servings of other fruits and vegetables. All these berries are high in potassium and vitamin C and protect against inflammation.

Apples are packed full of antioxidants, especially vitamin C for healthy skin and gums. Apples also contain a form of soluble fiber called pectin that can help lower blood cholesterol levels and can keep the digestive system healthy. An apple is also a carbohydrate with a low glycemic index (GI) type. Low GI foods are digested slowly; once the pectin has finally broken down in the intestine, it's slowly absorbed into the bloodstreams as glucose, causing a gradual rise in blood-sugar levels. This property can improve diabetics' ability to control their blood-sugar levels.

Avocados contain heart-healthy monounsaturated fat, which helps to reduce bad cholesterol and lower risk of illness and disease. Avocados also contain proteins and nutrients like folate and vitamin E, which makes them the best food to eat for a healthy complexion. Spread it on your face, or whip up a batch of guacamole.

Grapefruits, lemons, and oranges contain high concentrations of vitamin C, vitamin A, antioxidants, flavonoids, potassium, calcium, magnesium, and dietary fiber that make them superfoods. These citrus fruit are useful to aid in reducing bad cholesterol and lowering blood-pressure levels. Lemons and grapefruit help the liver eliminate toxins. Lemons also alkalize the blood and help cleanse the liver by stimulating the release of enzymes.

Fresh pineapple is rich in nutrients like vitamin C, manganese, and copper. Pineapples contain the enzyme bromelain, which helps with the digestion of protein, and they are also high in fiber.

Bananas are a good source of potassium and are helpful to your heart. They can deliver the energy needed after a long workout while fighting muscle cramps in the process. Bananas also have antacid effects, protecting the stomach from ulcers. Potassium is essential for muscle contraction. Low levels can cause cramps or spasms. Because the heart is a muscle, Vitamin K is essential for normal heart function.

Pears are anti-inflammatory, making them a great postworkout snack to ease your hard-working muscles. They also have lots of dietary fiber as well, which aids digestion. Pears also contain phytonutrients, which can potentially guard against cancer-causing carcinogens.

Pomegranates are rich in potassium, vitamin C, polyphenols, and vitamin B6, making them real phytochemical powerhouses. Pomegranate juice may have two to three times more antioxidant power than green tea or red wine. Pomegranates possess potent anti-inflammatory phytochemicals, and drinking pomegranate juice has been shown to lower blood pressure.

Healthy oils like primrose and flaxseed oil can help correct an out-of-balance pH when taken every day. Cod-liver oil and pumpkin-seed oil are incredibly rich in fat-soluble vitamins and other nutrients. Healthier alternatives to use in cooking are olive oil, avocado oil, and coconut oil, which is especially good for improving your skin and hair.

There are four basic types of fat that our bodies need, and we get them from our food choices. These fats are polyunsaturated, cholesterol, monounsaturated, and saturated. Polyunsaturated omega-3 fatty acids are essential to promote and maintain a good, healthy lifestyle. Due to the over processing of our foods and oils, we consume an abundance of omega-6 fatty acids and little to none of the omega-3 fatty acids. The typical Standard American Diet (SAD) is high in omega-6-rich foods like cereals, baked goods, fried foods, margarine, processed breads, and overly refined foods and oils.

The lack of omega-3 shows up in a multitude of disorders of the brain such as Alzheimer's, autism, ADD, ADHD, and depression. An easy fix is to add omega-3 rich foods to your diet like quality, raw flaxseed, borage, walnuts, pumpkin seed oils, and dark, leafy green vegetables to your plate, salad, or smoothie. These dietary changes can make a difference in your mental and physical health. These seed and nut oils are called short-chain fatty acids, while the fish oils are long-chain fatty acids.

Omega-3 oils have many health benefits, including improved heart health, easing of menstrual pain and PMS, improved insulin sensitivity for type-two diabetics, natural blood thinning properties that can help prevent strokes, reduced hypertension, lowered blood pressure levels, reduced autoimmune disease symptoms, help for arthritis and fatigue, improved depression and overall mental health. Omega-3 oils are most prevalent in fatty, cold-water fish. When buying fish, you want to look for wild (not farmed) salmon, sardines, mackerel, and herring. Try to eat two to three servings of fish per week. Omegas 3s are also found in eggs. You can ditch the egg-white-only mantra, by the way. Yolks contain the bulk of the egg's nutrients, including minerals like calcium and magnesium and vitamins A, D, E, B6, B12, and the list goes on! Eggs have 100 percent of the carotenoids essential for healthy eyes, protecting them against vision loss. Eggs are also rich in protein, and they are an energy-sustaining food that helps stave off fatigue.

Nuts and seeds are nutritional powerhouses and make a much better snack than prepackaged snacks. With a relatively high fat content, most nuts and seeds are satisfying and healthy foods that will diminish hunger and can actually help you lose weight. Choose organic nuts, such as almonds or walnuts and make your own butter by putting them into a food processor and pulsing.

Flaxseed is a good source of omega-3 fatty acids. Flaxseeds cleanse the digestive tract and help thin blood to reduce clotting. They are helpful with weight loss, and they rehydrate the skin from the inside. You can grind the seeds, sprinkle them on a salad, or put them into a smoothie.

Pumpkin seeds are great source of iron, zinc, and selenium. They help decrease skin inflammation.

Sesame seeds are high in iron and calcium. Black seeds and their oil are helpful to lubricate the heart, liver, kidneys, pancreas, and lungs. They are excellent for cleansing the colon. Sesamol, a compound found in sesame seeds and sesame oil, has been shown in some studies to protect against DNA damaged caused by radiation.

Walnuts are a great source of omega-3 fatty acids, and they lower cholesterol. They are a really good source of copper, which supports immune function. Walnut kernels can also help with healing inflammatory skin conditions like eczema.

Almonds reduce cholesterol and are a great source for calcium.

Hemp seeds are packed with pure digestible protein and are rich in amino acids, iron, and vitamin E, as well as omega-3's. Hemp is the perfect food if you're looking to increase protein. Get the benefit of omega-3's by lightly toasting hemp seeds in a skillet and sprinkling them on your food, or you can add these seeds to your smoothie.

Chia seeds are rich in antioxidants, vitamins, minerals, and fiber. This super seed also contains 500 percent more calcium than milk and the same amount of omega-3s as wild salmon. The same seed also has an appetite-suppressing quality, helping you feel full and making chia seeds an ideal food for your weight-loss program. They are also loaded with protein; I just love this seed.

Sunflower seeds are a great source of dietary fiber, protein, and complex carbohydrates. They prevent rheumatoid arthritis, aid in digestion, improve memory, and increase energy. Sunflower seeds are a great source of magnesium, which helps to strengthen bones, lower high blood pressure, prevent migraine headaches, and reduce the risk of heart attacks and strokes.

New supplements and herbs, such as maca, a root that belongs to the radish family and mangosteen, an East Indian fruit are being recognized and discovered each year.

Probiotics means "pro-life" while antibiotics means "against life." As beneficial as antibiotics have proven to be against bacterial infections, they also destroy the good intestinal flora in our gut. Problems arise after years of taking antibiotics and not replacing the good bacteria that has been lost. Probiotics, such as acidophilus and bifidobacteruim populate our intestinal tract. Their functions are very important for the effective breakdown, digestion, and absorption of vital nutrients. There are hundreds of different species of bacteria in our gut, but these two keep yeast and parasites under control. However, once the antibiotics wipe out the probiotics, yeast and parasites are free to grow and do so at an alarming rate. Consider some of the standard symptoms from an overgrowth of yeast in the system: bloating, indigestion, and constipation, itchy skin, diarrhea, nail fungus, weight gain, and fatigue.

Protein powders are highly concentrated forms of protein made from soy, whey, egg, rice, pea, hemp, or sprouted grains. During the mindful eating program I recommend, you can use rice protein powder or pea and egg protein in your morning smoothies. You can also add the egg protein to baked goods.

Maca increases energy, endurance, strength, and libido. Dried maca powder contains seven essential amino acids, twenty additional amino acids, and is 10 percent protein.

Blue green algae from the Upper Klamath Lake

What are the differences between Klamath Blue Green Algae (Aphanizomenon Flos Aquae or AFA), spirulina and chlorella. AFA and spirulina are blue green algaes while chlorella is a green algae, which means it has an indigestible cellulose wall. This wall must be mechanically broken in order for the body to be able to digest it.

Spirulina and chlorella are cultivated in man-made ponds whereas AFA is wildcrafted from Upper Klamath Lake where it grows in a pristine, mineral rich environment that cannot be duplicated synthetically. The difference in energy one receives from these whole foods is similar to the difference between cultivated produce and foraged wild vegetables and fruits.

Spirulina and Chlorella are usually heat processed for commercial distribution. The cell walls of Spirulina are carmelized during spray drying, making it difficult for enzymes to penetrate the algae cells during digestion. This results in low assimilation of proteins and other nutritional components. Spray drying can also kill enzymes, losing heat sensitive components and decreasing beta-carotene due to the high temperatures that may be involved.

AFA blue-green algae, is the most complete protein and has a vast array of minerals, phytonutrients, and enzymes. According to Christian Drapeau in his book *Primordial Food*, AFA blue-green algae increases our internal production of stem cells. You can add this super supplement right to your smoothies or shakes; it's awesome! It's also a great supplement if you want healthy, strong hair.

Bee products have many health benefits. Bee pollen is one of the most complete foods found in nature, containing nearly all the B vitamins, especially B9 (folate), and all twenty-one essential amino acids—making it a complete protein. It can be taken as a supplement or put right into your shakes or smoothies. Honey, in its organic, raw state, is rich with minerals, antioxidants, probiotics, and enzymes. For maximum health benefits, raw, local honey should be used.

Mangosteen, not related to the mango, has an abundance of phytonutrients called xanthones, which are super antioxidants known for their potency. Its anti-inflammatory properties help repair cellular damage that causes neurological pain and discomfort. Dr. John Edwards gives you seventy-three more reasons why you should drink mangosteen. It can be purchased in powder form or as a liquid. Dr. Edwards book "The Mangosteen Revolution", offers an extensive overview of the history of the Mangosteen fruit, its traditional uses, health benefits, and how it works once inside the human body and on the cellular level. Dr. John Edwards covers the following health topics: obesity, diabetes, high blood pressure, weight loss, & cholesterol problems. His second book covers the leukemia's, autoimmune diseases like lupus, rheumatoid arthritis, parkinson's, alzheimer's, autism, ADHD, schizophrenia, and bipolar disorder.

Vegetable superfoods include many of the veggies that you may find on your dinner plate regularly—such as broccoli, pumpkin, and carrots—but there are also some more unusual options like shiitake mushrooms and sweet potatoes. All of these vegetables are very valuable nutritionally and well worth eating often.

Artichokes lower uric-acid levels. They also contain compounds that assist in the production and elimination of bile, which is the fluid discharge of toxins that the liver produces. Sufficient bile production helps to ensure that toxins are efficiently removed from the body.

Red beets have unusually high nitrate levels, which helps reduce blood pressure. Virtually fat free and rich in iron and magnesium content, beets may help to treat anemia and tiredness. They are also rich in folic acid, which is known to reduce the risks of birth defects if taken before conception and during the early stages of pregnancy. The rich color of beets comes from betalains, a cancer-fighting phytonutrient. Besides their liver-protecting qualities, beets also dilate the body's vessels so blood flows more easily. They also contain iron, which helps deliver oxygen throughout the body and fights anemia.

Sweet potatoes are rich in beta-carotene and antioxidants and are also super high in heart-healthy vitamin A. They're packed with vitamin C to keep your immune system strong, and are an excellent food choice for those suffering from arthritis or asthma. People with diabetes may also benefit from eating this root vegetable because it ranks low on the glycemic index and has less of an effect on blood-glucose levels.

Seaweed and sea vegetables have tremendous health benefits. They contain nutrients that help to remove heavy metals and detoxify the body. They also provide minerals that can regulate cholesterol.

Seaweed benefits the entire body, and it is especially excellent for the thyroid, immune system, adrenals, and hormone function.

Medicinal mushrooms like reishi, maitake, shiitake, and lion's mane contain super immune-enhancing components. They have also been proven effective in fighting off cancer cells. You can purchase them in powdered form or in capsules, as well as dried or fresh mushrooms.

Artichokes have a diuretic effect on the kidneys while helping to cleanse the liver of toxins. They help to restore and promote the flow of bile from the gallbladder for better digestion of fats.

Broccoli is high in phytonutrients and iron and has cleansing properties. By cleansing, we essentially "heal" the body from the inside, out, allowing for bodily rejuvenation all the way down to a cellular level.

Celery is loaded with antioxidants. It has amazing diuretic properties and is especially beneficial to the kidneys. Celery lowers uric-acid levels in the blood, which reduces the risk of developing kidney stones.

Carrots are helpful for stimulating the elimination of wastes from the intestines. They are also a rich source of beta-carotene.

Dandelion is a good source of iron and copper. Its diuretic properties help in the treatment of high blood pressure and water retention. Dandelion is also helpful for cleansing and strengthening the liver.

Green leafy vegetables are the best source of alkaline minerals and fiber and have many calming, antistress properties. They are also the best source of chlorophyll. Chlorophyll is a blood builder and is one of the most abundant foods on earth. Spinach, kale, alfalfa, spirulina, chlorella, blue-green algae, collard greens, Swiss chard, watercress, arugula, wheat grass, and lettuces are all great examples of delicious greens.

Mustard greens are spicy greens that are rich in vitamin K and are good for your blood and for your bone strength. They're also rich in natural substances called sulforaphanes that, when eaten, help the body get rid of bile acid from the gut. The body uses bile acids to make cholesterol, so less bile acid results in less cholesterol.

Kale is high in the nutrients iron, calcium, and beta-carotene. It stimulates the immune system and eases lung congestion.

Asparagus, cauliflower, and cabbage are full of sulfur and glutathione. These foods help in the cleansing process, especially when eaten raw.

Grains and Beans

Quinoa is a grain that is considered to be a perfect protein, containing nine essential amino acids. It contains twice the fiber of most grains, and it helps to lower cholesterol and to keep your heart healthy.

Brown rice helps to cleanse the intestines by providing fiber. It can be used to treat the nervous system and depression. It is a good source of potassium and magnesium.

Black Rice is even better for you than brown rice. That's because the bran hull contains significantly higher amounts of vitamin E, which bolsters the immune system and protects cells from free-radical damage.

Vitamins and Minerals

Vitamin A is found in fish oils, egg yolk, liver, and beta carotene (which is found in yellow and orange vegetables and fruits).
It is needed for healthy eyes, including night vision.

Vitamins B1–6 are found in nuts, sunflower seeds, eggs, almonds, green leafy vegetables, seafood, beans, and liver.
It is needed for a healthy nervous system, healthy hair, skin, and nails, hormone production, and muscles.

Vitamin B12 is found in liver, oily fish, and egg yolks.
It is needed to prevent infection and to prevent mental deterioration in old age.

Vitamin C is found in fresh fruits and vegetables.
It is needed to prevent infection and heart disease.

Vitamin D is found in green, leafy vegetables, mushrooms, eggs, milk, and butter.
It is needed for a healthy heart and nervous system.

Vitamin E is found in wheat germ oil, nuts, seeds, and whole grains.
It is needed for healthy cell membranes, fertility, stamina, and combating the changes of old age.

Folic acid is found in leafy, green vegetables, fruits, whole grains, milk, and liver.
It is needed to prevent heart disease, birth abnormalities, and anemia.

Minerals
Calcium is found in green, leafy vegetables, seeds, and nuts.
It is needed for healthy bones, teeth, and muscles.

Chromium is found in egg yolks, molasses, red meat, wine, whole grains, and vegetables.
It is needed to maintain the correct blood-sugar levels and cholesterol.

Iodine is found in fish and sea vegetables.
It is needed for the thyroid glands to function effectively.

Iron is found in liver, red meat, whole grains, beans, and green vegetables.
It is needed to prevent anemia.

Magnesium is found in nuts, whole grains, fruit, and green vegetables.

It is needed for normal muscle function and blood pressure, to prevent fatigue.

Potassium is found in fruits, vegetables, salmon, and lamb.
It is needed for healthy bones and to combat fatigue and muscle weakness.

Zinc is found in seafood, whole grains, nuts, and seeds.
It is needed to fight infection, repair wounds, and for normal sexual function.

TO GO ORGANIC OR NOT? THAT IS THE QUESTION.

*O*rganic refers to a way in which food is grown, raised, or produced. Originally, all foods were "organic." They were grown and prepared without pesticides, herbicides, chemical fertilizers, hormones, or irradiation. Foods were unrefined, whole, or minimally processed. After World War II, the factories that were making weapons began to make chemicals for farming and food processing, and now the soil and foods of much of our world have been depleted of important minerals and nutrients.

The food we are eating now, whether it is vegetable or animal protein, is not only deficient in nutrients, but it is full of chemicals and pesticides. Pesticides, which have been shown to cause cancer and diseases of the liver, kidney, and blood, create extra work for the immune system. In addition, as pesticides build up in our tissues, they weaken our immune system allowing other carcinogens and pathogens to affect our health.

Getting back to organic farming that works the land means crops are rotated from year to year in order to allow the soil to regain nutrients between growing cycles. Animals feed from the land as well. The farmer fertilizes the soil with a compost of manure, rather than using toxic fertilizers. These practices are a long-term, sustainable method of farming that works with the natural environment, instead of adding chemicals.

Here are the top reasons to buy organic and to eat organically.

1. Chemicals—Pesticides are poison designed to kill living organisms. Many approved pesticides were registered long before extensive research linked these chemicals to cancer and other diseases. Organic agriculture is a way to prevent any more of these chemicals from getting into the air, water, and food supply.

2. Protect future generations—Children are four times more sensitive to exposure from cancer-causing pesticides in foods than adults.

3. Protect water quality—Pesticides pollute more than half the country's primary source of drinking water.

4. Save energy-—More energy is now used to produce synthetic fertilizers than to till, cultivate, and harvest all the crops in the United States.

5. Support local economy—Organic foods may appear to be expensive at first. However, keep in mind that your tax dollars pay for hazardous waste cleanup and environmental damage caused by conventional farming. If we can depend more on organic produce, we can lower the amount of damage that we have to pay to clean up.

Many people may not be able to buy organic all the time; you don't have to buy all organic produce to reduce the risk of chemical contamination. This list from the Environmental Working Group shows us which fruits and vegetables contain the most chemicals and which ones are least contaminated. Use it when you're shopping to make the best choices on buying organic or nonorganic.

Dirty Dozen Plus (Produce with the most pesticides, in order from the most contaminated)

Try to grow these organically yourself.

1. Apples
2. Celery
3. Strawberries
4. Peaches
5. Spinach
6. Nectarines (imported)
7. Grapes
8. Sweet bell peppers
9. Kale/Collard greens
10. Hot peppers
11. Cherries
12. Tomatoes
13. Summer squash/Zucchini
14. Cucumbers
15. Potatoes

Clean Fifteen (Produce with the least amount of pesticides, in order from the least contaminated)

1. Onions
2. Pineapple
3. Avocado
4. Asparagus
5. Corn

6. Sweet peas (frozen)
7. Mango
8. Eggplant
9. Cantaloupe
10. Kiwi
11. Cabbage
12. Watermelon
13. Sweet potatoes
14. Grapefruit
15. Mushrooms
16. Papayas

If you are going to the store, and you're going to buy any of the dirty dozen, at least you should arm yourself with a solution and a vegetable brush that will help you clean your produce to remove those nasty pesticides so that they don't become part of you and your cellular tissues. When you get home from the grocery store, clean your produce before you put it away. It takes about ten minutes to clean and prep fruits and vegetables for the week.

Mix one part white vinegar to three parts water. The exact proportion doesn't matter. Soak the produce in the water-vinegar mixture for about two minutes. Put all your fruits and vegetables in the bath, or separate them, if you prefer. Wash the firmer-skinned produce, like your apples and peppers, with the vegetable brush. Rinse well under water for thirty seconds. You must look at the solution before and after you wash your produce. You will be glad you bought this book for that reason alone when you see how dirty the water looks.

Organic, healthy whole foods are grown without hormones and pesticides. They are not processed, and they do not contain refined sugar. Shop on the outside perimeter of the grocery store where you can find whole fruits and vegetables, nuts, and seeds. Eating whole fruits and vegetables within a day of when they are picked will provide the most nutritional benefits. Frozen whole fruits and vegetables can also be a nutritious choice; they are flash frozen as soon as they are picked.

One more reason to eat organic is to avoid genetically modified organisms (GMOs). GMOs are any organism in which the genetic material has been altered or shuffled around in a way that does not occur naturally. The most common genetically engineered crops in the United States, which is the largest grower of GM crops in the world, are canola, corn, soy, and cotton. Genetically engineered soy, corn, and canola are used in many processed foods; the government does not require labeling of these foods. Many experts estimate that about 70 percent of the foods in the grocery stores in the United States and Canada contain genetically engineered ingredients. To avoid them, look for labels that say "GMO free" or Organic.

Food-Label Claims

Now I am going to share with you a section-by-section guide to the best and worst foods in your grocery store. Many food labels can be confusing, so knowing what a food claim truly means is a great way to educate yourself about where your food comes from and how it has been produced. New food-label claims arise regularly, so, if you come across a new phrase, be sure to take time to do your own research and learn what it really means.

Meat and Dairy Section

Look for the labels USDA-Certified Organic, Animal-Welfare Approved, Certified Human and Global Animal Partnership.

Avoid food with the labels Natural, Free-Range, Cage-Free, and Hormone-Free. Also avoid flavored milk and "light" or "lite" products.

Natural—There are currently no standards for this label except when used on meat and poultry products. The USDA guidelines state that "natural" meat and poultry products can only undergo minimal processing and cannot contain artificial ingredients. However, foods labeled "natural" are not necessarily raised on a sustainable farm, organic, humanely raised, or free of hormones and antibiotics.

Cage-free—This means that the birds are raised without cages. What this doesn't explain is whether the birds were raised outdoors on pasture or if they were raised indoors in overcrowded conditions. If you are looking to buy eggs, poultry, or meat that was raised outdoors, look for labels that say "pastured" or "pasture-raised."

Free-range—The terms "free-range" or "free-roaming" are only defined by the USDA for egg and poultry production. The label can be used as long as the producers allow the birds access to the outdoors so that they can engage in natural behaviors. It doesn't necessarily mean that the products are cruelty-free or antibiotic-free or that the animals spent the majority of their time outdoors. Claims are defined by the USDA but are not verified by third-party inspectors.

Hormone-Free—The USDA has prohibited the use of the term "hormone-free," but animals that were raised without added growth hormones can be labeled "no hormones administered" or "no added hormones." By law hogs and poultry cannot be given any hormones. If the meats you are buying are not clearly labeled, ask your farmer or butcher if they are free from hormones.

Bakery

Look for 100% whole wheat or 100% whole grains.

Avoid the label "Made with Whole Grains."

Processed Foods

Look for the label "No trans fats." Also look for products that contain four grams of saturated fat or less, six hundred milligrams of sodium or less, five hundred total calories or less, and four grams of sugar or less.

Avoid diacetyl, which is an artificial butter flavor, artificial sweeteners, sugar alcohols, high-fructose corn syrup, brown-rice syrup, and hydrogenated anything.

Produce

Whether you're shopping organic or trying to avoid genetically modified foods, the PLU label on your produce can tell you what you're buying.

A five-digit number that starts with a 9 means the item *is* organic.

A four-digit number that starts with a 3 or a 4 means the item is conventionally grown.

A five-digit number that starts with an 8 means the item is genetically modified.

An "**Organic**" designation means that all organic agriculture farms and products must meet the following guidelines (verified by a USDA-approved, independent agency).

1. Abstain from the application of prohibited materials (including synthetic fertilizers, pesticides, and sewage sludge) for three years prior to certification and then continually throughout the organic licensing period.
2. Prohibit the use of genetically modified organisms and irradiation.

3. Employ positive soil-building, conservation, manure-management, and crop-rotation practices.
4. Provide outdoor access and pasture for livestock.
5. Free of antibiotic and hormone use in animals.
6. Sustain animals on 100 percent organic feed.
7. Avoid contamination during the processing of organic products.
8. Keep records of all operations.

If a product has the "USDA Organic" seal, it means that 95–100 percent of its ingredients are organic. Products with 70–95 percent organic ingredients can still advertise "organic ingredients" on the front of the package, and products with less than 70 percent organic ingredients can identify the organic ingredients on the side panel. Organic foods prohibit the use of hydrogenation and trans fats.

The "Fair-Trade" label means that farmers and workers, who are often in developing countries, have received a fair wage and worked in acceptable conditions while growing and packaging the product.

What Does Mindful Eating Mean?

*M*indful eating means eating with awareness. So often many of us mindlessly stuff food into our mouths while we are sitting in front of the television or computer, while we are driving, or while running out of the house.

Mindful eating is a process where you can eat what you love, enjoy it completely, slow down, and fully experience all the elements of the food you are putting into your mouth.

There are many elements to mindful eating, so just pick one, and try it. Add a second element the next time you are eating, then add a third until you are completely conscious about what you are eating. It's all about making small changes to create healthy, new habits.

You can also start this plan with another person; the important part is to have fun creating new, healthy habits. It's a simple commitment to be grateful, appreciative, and respectful, and to enjoy the food we eat every day. Mindful eating can be practiced any time you eat; you can introduce the new healthy habit at home, at work, or even eating a snack, while on the go.

Sight—Look at your food; really check it out. Can you imagine how the food was hydrated? What type of water do you think nourished the food? Was it rain? Can you see the sunlight within the food? Notice the bright, beautiful colors and the way the food is arranged on the plate.

Smell—Bring the food up to your nose; experience smelling the food. Is it hot? Can you smell the aroma of the food, the herbs and the spices? Is it cold? Does it have the crisp smell of fresh vegetables? Maybe it doesn't have a smell.

Taste—Can you feel your mouth starting to produce saliva as you anticipate the food going into your mouth? How does the food feel in your mouth? Give all your attention to your mouth and chewing. Notice which side of your mouth the food is going on. Take your time and enjoy your food; it's very healthy to do this. Eat slowly; it's not race. Try to chew the food twenty to thirty times before you swallow. Your digestive system will have a much easier time breaking down the food. Eating with chopsticks is a great way to slow down; there are beginner chopsticks, in case you need them.

I remember when I was a kid, my mother said, "Let's see who can chew their food the longest." I always won. I was always the last one at the table. I just loved to chew the flavors out of the food. That may sound weird, and I didn't know why then, but I do now.

Pay attention to the flavors and textures of the food while it's in your mouth. Does it have a citrus, sweet, earthy, spicy, creamy, or grilled flavor? Does it have a smooth, chunky, or liquid texture?

Be silent.—Take some simple steps to have quieter meals and snacks. This can be as easy as silencing your cell phones and shutting off television to eat dinner or turning off the music in the car.

I remember another thing my mother would say while we were at the dinner/supper table was, "Let's see who can eat without talking for five minutes." I somehow lost that one a lot.

If you feeling much too busy for a meal? Or too much stress/busyness in life, you can simply sip tea silently.

Feel—Mindful eating happens when you pay attention to how the food is making you feel. Eating can be an experience with each bite. Eating mindful has all of the sensory experiences associated with it: sexy, beautiful, stimulating, and healthy. Your body knows when to stop eating so you can maintain a healthy weight. There are plenty of easy ways to work mindfulness into new healthy daily habits

Mindfulness is having a relationship with our food. Plant yourself a vegetable or herb garden, or visit a working farm. (This is an ideal place to get nutritious whole foods.) Go to a farmer's market, and check out their produce; usually it's just been picked. Go to the grocery store or health-food store, and look at the produce and products.

Look for community-supported agriculture (CSA). In CSAs the farmer offers a certain number of shares to the public. The share consists of a box of vegetables, but other farm products may be included. Each week you pick up your share of vegetables at the farm. This arrangement creates several rewards for both the farmer and the consumer. The advantages for the consumer include the ability to eat local and ultra-fresh food with the entire flavor and nutritional benefits of just-picked vegetables, exposure to new vegetables and new ways of cooking, the opportunity to develop a relationship with the farmers, and the chance to learn more about how food is grown. The advantages for the farmer include the opportunity to get to know the people who eat the food they grow and payment early in the season, which helps with the farm's cash flow.

A locavore is a person who prefers to eat food grown or produced with a one-hundred-mile radius of home. Buying locally grown produce and products is an excellent idea. You can't beat the taste of a fresh local tomato or a freshly picked strawberry. Buying local also plays an important role in preserving farmland in your area.

Think about the origins of your food, even if you have no idea where the food you're eating has come from. Ask yourself questions about the possibilities: Where did it come from? Who grew it? How did it get here? You will have a greater appreciation and connection to the food you put into your body.

Be mindful of what you are putting in your mouth. If you try one new, healthy habit a week or a month, you will develop truly lasting, healthy lifestyle habits. Try it! It's easy and fun.

"A Rainbow of Foods"

E nergy comes from the nourishment of foods we eat and lifestyle choices we make.

Foods we eat can either increase our energy or decrease our energy. Increase you energy by making changes in your diet. Increase your morning calorie intake, decrease your evening calorie intake, and incorporate quality protein, eating it first at every meal.

Eating more whole foods is our best bet for improving health and preventing disease. Eating a rainbow of food colors promotes DNA health, protects and produces cells on a cellular level, improves the immune system, supports brain health, decreases inflammation, and protects our hearts.

A natural, beautiful bright-orange or red color in food is a good indicator that it is rich in lycopene, which is a powerful antioxidant. Foods that fall in this category include fresh tomatoes, watermelon, grapefruit, cooked red cabbage, guava, papayas, cooked red peppers, mango, and sun-dried tomatoes,

A food that is high in lycopene but is not orange or red in color is cooked asparagus, and dried basil

Resveratrol, found in the skin of red grapes and red wine, is a member of a group of plant compounds called polyphenols. These compounds are thought to have antioxidant properties that neutralize free radicals linked to increased risk for conditions such as cancer and heart disease. Resveratrol is found in other sources include peanuts and berries. The vitality of the color orange is reflected in vitamin-C rich oranges and tangerines. The beta-carotene in these fruits also converts to vitamin A, which is good for your eyes and promotes a healthy immune system, as well as bone and cellular growth. Other orange foods with these properties include carrots, pumpkin, cantaloupe, papaya, sweet potatoes, and winter squash.

Foods that are not orange but are high in vitamin A and beta-carotene are spinach, collard greens, kale, cabbage, beets, and turnip greens.

Yellow foods play a vital role in the energy system of the body. These foods contain vitamin C and include yellow bell peppers, lemons, and grapefruit—which also helps the liver to eliminate toxins. Citrus may lower cholesterol and protect against some cancers. Fresh pineapple contains bromelain, which helps with the digestion of protein.

Food exceptions that are not yellow but that are loaded with vitamin C are kiwi, broccoli, strawberries, peas, and guava.

Green foods are the most vital of all the other foods we eat. Chlorophyll is the nutrient found in these foods that reduces our risk for chronic illness, lowers blood pressure, supports eye health and vision, fights free radicals, and boosts our immune system. These foods can be very supportive and cleansing. They include celery, cucumbers, brussels sprouts, avocado, leeks, green beans, kale, arugula, chard, collard greens, watercress, and all dark leafy vegetables.

Leafy greens keep eyes strong, protecting the retina and reducing the risk of cataracts and age-related degeneration.

Blue and purple foods are good for brain memory and function. They help reduce the risk of stroke and heart disease, and they support cardiovascular health as we age. Purple foods play a significant role in healing the mind and balancing the nervous system. These foods include blueberries, purple grapes, blackberries, purple cabbage, purple cauliflower, purple plums, figs, prunes, and raisins. Black rice is also a must to try, as it has more antioxidants than blueberries.

White foods are very helpful for the heart and prevent chronic illness. These foods are bananas, cauliflower, garlic, mushrooms, and beans (black, red, white, and yellow).

CHAPTER TWO

HAVE YOU CHECKED YOUR PH TODAY?

The body's pH balance is extremely important indicator to use to maintain a healthy lifestyle and essential for a happy life. What is pH? The symbol pH stands for potential, or power, of hydrogen, which is a measurement of the hydrogen ion concentration in the body. The pH scale ranges from one to fourteen, with seven considered to be neutral. A pH of less than seven is acidic, and a pH greater than seven is alkaline. You can test your pH levels regularly by dipping a piece of litmus paper in your saliva or urine first thing in the morning before eating or drinking anything.

The body is largely made up of water, which transports nutrients, oxygen, and biochemicals from place to place inside your body. Since the body is water based, the pH level has profound effects on all body chemistry, health, and disease. If your pH is too acidic or too alkaline, cells become poisoned by their own toxic waste and die. When body tissues have a balanced pH level, it makes it easier for the cells to discard waste and toxins.

Is an imbalanced body pH really dangerous?

The short answer is, yes. Healthy living cells do not do well in an overly acidic or overly alkaline environment. Just like acid rain can destroy a forest and alkaline waste pollutes a lake, an imbalanced overly acidic pH continuously corrodes all body tissue, slowly eating into the thousands and thousands of miles of our veins and arteries like corrosives eating into marble. As a person is growing up, this condition may go undetected. An imbalanced pH can lead to most fatal diseases: cardiovascular disease (the number one killer in the United States), cancer (the number two killer in the United States), diabetes, and obesity, which both have a very disturbing growth rate in the United States.

It makes sense that a highly acidic pH encourages the growth of cancer cells and tumors. By eating mostly foods that help balance the body's pH there is less of a chance that cancer cells will develop and grow. When you adjust the way you eat, you can actually improve your chance of experiencing good health. Cancer cells do not grow in the presence of oxygen, but when oxygen levels are low, cancer cells have an opportunity to multiply.

What causes pH to become imbalanced?

What people put into their mouths can cause an unhealthy pH. Addressing an acidic or alkaline imbalance is fundamental to bringing the body back to balance and health.

Here are nine reasons why you should check your pH balance.

1) A balanced pH allows the digestive system to achieve proper fat metabolism, weight control, and healthy insulin production. Most digestive disorders such as nausea, bloating, and gastric reflux are symptoms caused by excess acid in the gastric region and not enough alkaline minerals in the intestinal tract. If the

alkaline minerals from enzyme-rich foods are missing, then the pancreas will become exhausted and will lose the ability to break down food and tell the body what to do with it. This will lead to inflammation.

2) A balanced pH allows the circulatory system to maintain proper blood-pressure regulation. When the body has an acidic pH, arteries become dilated, which makes the heart work overtime. It is well established that many fats are extremely important and essential for cardiovascular health. Good fats can actually help heal inflammation. When the arteries thicken with plaque, it is not a response to good fats. It is inflammation created by factors like poor diet, high blood pressure, diabetes, obesity and stress that make an internal body system an acidic environment. The body then responds to the acidity by lining the vessels with fatty plaques to prevent life-threatening leaks. This, in turn, strains the heart because the aperture (opening) for the blood to flow through is narrower. When the heart becomes completely exhausted, this is known as a heart attack.

3) A balanced pH allows the respiratory system to sustain a healthy oxygen flow to tissues to flush toxins and protect against premature aging. When the tissues and organs are overloaded by acidity, the transport of oxygen is strangled. This suffocation means normal healthy cells cannot breathe properly. Every cell in our body needs to breathe new oxygen and to clear acidic carbon dioxide in order to function correctly. When the acidity is too high, infections and viruses build up in our lung, which can lead to colds, bronchitis, and asthma.

4) A balanced pH allows proper calcium utilization, which in turn lessens the possibility of osteoporosis and arthritis. Arthritis is one of the most disabling diseases. The word arthritis means "inflammation of the joint" and is used to describe pain,

stiffness, and swelling in the joints. The two main forms of arthritis are rheumatoid and osteoarthritis. Both forms are related to pH imbalance and accumulation of acid deposits in the joints and wrists. It is this accumulated acid that damages cartilage. When the cells that produce the lubricating fluids are acidic, they do not do their job properly. This causes a dryness that irritates and swells the joints. When uric acid builds up, it tends to create deposits in the form of crystals, which feel like broken glass in the feet, hands, knees, and back. Some arthritis can be reversed with a specific protocol using alkaline minerals and yoga.

5) A balanced pH allows proper kidney function. The excretory system is also known as the urinary system. It is made up of multiple organs, the main one being the kidneys. The kidneys perform the task of filtering fluids and purifying the blood. If excess acids overwhelm the body, alkaline minerals are pulled from our bones and dumped in the blood. If this occurs frequently enough, the minerals build up in the kidneys in the form of kidney stones.

6) A balanced pH allows proper electrolyte activity in the nervous system. An acidic body weakens the nervous system by depriving it of energy. It makes the body emotionally, mentally, and physically weak.

7) A balanced pH allows cellular regeneration and DNA synthesis within the immune system. Acidic environments are breeding grounds for pathogens (free radicals), which are high levels of hydrogen. Whether bad bacteria and free radicals incubate or remain dormant all depends on the ratio of cellular pH. Free radicals range from cancerous cells to cellular mutations. For DNA synthesis and the body's natural

cleansing and healing processes to occur, cellular pH cannot be acidic.

8) A balanced pH allows access to energy reserves in the muscular system. When acidity increases in the muscle cells, it disrupts the metabolism breakdown of glucose and oxygen to energy. This means muscles perform poorly in an acidic environment. An alkaline system, on the other hand, allows for much better aerobic metabolism and energy for the body's recovery. When someone's body is acidic, that person breathes by taking large gulping inhales while doing the simplest tasks, like walking and talking. This is because an acidic body finds it difficult to deliver oxygen to the cells.

9) There's a lot of research being done on our reproductive system to discover the exact link between sexual dysfunction and infertility and a body with an acidic pH. An acidic person has a decrease in arousal, sexual enjoyment, and fertility and has an increased tendency to miscarry.

There are many more diseases and disorders that are associated with an acidic condition: cataracts, gout, cancer, migraines, constipation, morning sickness, stroke, allergies, diabetes, obesity, and more. With this awareness of how acidity affects us, we can all choose to be informed and empowered by making healthy decisions for a healthy lifestyle.

To check your pH, you can go to your local pharmacy or drug store to buy litmus paper. Test your saliva or urine first thing in the morning before eating or drinking. Check the color against the chart. On the next page, look at the chart of foods that you need to eat more of to balance your pH. This chart determines the effect the food has on the body after it has been consumed.

It might be a surprise that many fruits are considered acid forming. This is because of their high sugar content.

You may also have assumed that lemons and limes would be considered acidic; however, they both have a high-alkaline mineral content and almost no sugar. So after they are consumed, they have an alkaline effect on the body. Tomatoes also act the same way.

Soy sauce, miso, and tamari are fermented foods that are acid forming. This doesn't apply to the unfermented versions, and soy sauce and tofu are all right to consume as part of the 20 percent of mildly acidic foods that you are allowed to eat in your mindful-eating program.

Tea and coffee are acid forming. All herbal teas are alkaline, except for the fruity ones. Green tea has nearly as much caffeine as coffee, which makes it acid forming. However, if you merely want to reduce your caffeine intake, you may want to substitute green tea for coffee as your morning pick-me-up beverage. Rooibos tea is a great alternative; it's packed with antioxidants too.

White flour, white bread, pastries and pasta are all acid forming and tough to give up. Try sprouted breads, or even go for a wrap instead of a sandwich. Look for yeast free/gluten free varieties.

Understanding pH Levels and Why Many People Have Cancer and Other Diseases

If you have health problems, this is a sign that you are acidic. When the body goes into extreme acidosis, the kidneys start producing ammonia, which may cause the pH to test too alkaline. Treating for acidosis will help the kidneys to stop producing ammonia.

In 1960's only one person in two-hundred fourteen contracted cancer. Today cancer strikes one in three females and one out of every two males. The determining factor between health and disease is pH. It is not uncommon for the average American to test between four to five on the pH scale. Since oxygen levels in the body are directly related to pH, increasing pH from four to five increases the oxygen delivered to the cells by tenfold. Increasing the pH from four to six increases the oxygen one hundred times, and raising pH from four to seven increases oxygen levels one thousand times.

Research shows that unless the body's pH level is slightly alkaline, the body cannot heal itself. So no matter what type of modality you use to take care of your health problem, it won't be effective until the pH level is up. Most drugs, medications, and toxic chemicals have the effect of lowering the pH of the body.

When body pH drops below 6.4, enzymes are deactivated, digestion does not work properly, and vitamins, minerals, and food supplements cannot effectively assimilate. Acid decreases energy production in the cells, the ability to repair damaged cells, and the ability to detoxify heavy metals. It also makes the body more susceptible to fatigue and illness. Your body pH affects almost everything.

Research has proven that disease cannot survive in an alkaline state; however, viruses, bacteria, yeast, mold, fungus, candida, and cancer cells thrive in a low-oxygen, acidic-pH environment. An acidic pH can result from an acid-forming diet, emotional stress, toxic overload, immune reactions, or any process that deprives the cells of oxygen and other nutrients. The body will try to compensate for too much acid by using alkaline minerals, like sodium from the stomach and calcium from the bones. This is the cause of osteoporosis and a number of other diseases. If there are not enough minerals in the diet to compensate, a buildup of acids in the cells will occur, resulting in symptoms like pain, arthritis, fibromyalgia, multiple sclerosis, lupus, and others.

There are two factors that are *always* present with cancer no matter what else may be present. Those two factors are an acidic pH and lack of oxygen. Can we manipulate those two factors that are required for cancer to develop, and by doing so will that help reverse the cancer? If so we need to learn how to manipulate pH and oxygen.

Remember that the pH number is an exponent number of ten; therefore, a small difference in pH translates to a big difference in the number of oxygen (or OH) ions. In other words blood with a pH value of 7.45 contains 64.9 percent more oxygen than blood with a pH value of 7.3. Cancer needs an acidic, low-oxygen environment to survive and flourish. Terminal cancer patients are about one thousand times more acidic than they should be. This equates to dangerously low amounts of oxygen at the cellular level.

In the absence of oxygen, glucose undergoes fermentation to lactic acid. This causes the pH of the cell to drop even lower. The urine and saliva pH of terminal cancer patients almost always runs between 4.0 and 5.5. When the cancer goes into metastases, the pH drops even lower. Our bodies simply cannot fight disease if our body pH is not properly balanced. In other words it's either alkalize or die. It's that important!

Karen Mayo

Certified Nutrition Health and Lifestyle Coach

The At-A-Glance Acid/Alkaline Food List

EAT MORE →

← EAT LESS

↓ CAN BE INCLUDED IN YOUR 20% ACID ↓

Highly Alkaline	Moderately Alkaline	Mildly Alkaline	Neutral/Mildly Acidic	Moderately Acidic	Highly Acidic
pH 9.5 alkaline water	Avocado	Artichokes	Black Beans	Fresh, Natural Juice	Alcohol
Himalayan salt	Beetroot	Asparagus	Chickpeas/Garbanzos	Ketchup	Coffee
Grasses	Capsicum/Pepper	Brussells Sprouts	Kidney Beans	Mayonnaise	Fruit Juice (Sweetened)
Cucumber	Cabbage	Cauliflower	Seitan	Butter	Black Tea
Kale	Celery	Carrot	Cantaloupe	Apple	Cocoa
Spinach	Collard/Spring Greens	Chives	Currants	Apricot	Honey
Parsley	Endive	Courgette/Zuccini	Fresh Dates	Banana	Jam
Broccoli	Garlic	Leeks	Nectarine	Blackberry	Jelly
Sprouts (soy, alfalfa, etc.)	Ginger	New Baby Potatoes	Plum	Blueberry	Mustard
Sea Vegetables (Kelp)	Green Beans	Rhubarb	Sweet Cherry	Cranberry	Rice Syrup
Green drinks	Lettuce	Swede	Watermelon	Grapes	Soy Sauce
	Mustard Greens	Watercress	Amaranth	Mango	Vinegar
	Okra	Grapefruit	Millet	Orange	Yeast
	Onion	Coconut	Freshwater/Wild Fish	Peach	Dried Fruit
	Radish	Buckwheat	Rice Milk	Strawberry	Beef
	Red Onion	Quinoa	Soy Milk	Brown Rice	Chicken
	Rocket/Arugula	Spelt	Brazil Nuts	Oats	Eggs
	Tomato	Lentils	Pecan Nuts	Rye Bread	Farmed Fish
	Lemon	Tofu	Hazel Nuts	Wheat	Pork
	Lime	Goat Milk	Sunflower Oil	Wholemeal Bread	Shellfish
	Butter Beans	Most Herbs & Spices	Grapeseed Oil	Wild Rice	Cheese
	Soy Beans	Avocado Oil		Wholemeal Pasta	Dairy
	White Haricot Beans	Coconut Oil		Ocean Fish	Artificial Sweeteners
		Flax Oil			Syrup
		Udo's Oil			Mushroom

CHAPTER THREE

DO YOU HAVE THE SUGAR BLUES?

Conversations about sugar and the aging connection are always interesting. Some people are amazed at how much sugar they actually consume every day.

Sugar and caffeine are both highly addictive—so much so that the allure of Oreo cookies is being compared to cocaine or heroin. That's pretty serious, right? Let's look at a scenario that most people live every day. (I certainly used to when I worked in lending and finance.) It all starts in the morning with coffee and sugar or sugar substitute. Then we have another pick-me-up mid-morning. I would go to the vending machine or eat a chocolate bar at my desk. Then lunch was whatever everyone else was doing—processed foods full of sugar, salt and fat. Example of my lunch would be sandwiches, pizza, chips, and a soda. Then I had a second cup of coffee with sugar or sugar substitute or another trip to the vending machine. After work I had something to munch on before dinner. I ate dinner, filled with who knows what, at a restaurant. (Actually I can tell you, but you might not want to know. Google "meat glue.") Then there was dessert and another cup of coffee with sugar or sugar substitute. People wonder why others are so tired and irritable. It's because most of us have been caught in a cycle of riding the sugar roller coaster up then crashing. It's called the sugar blues; do you have them?

American's are the largest consumers of sugars, artificial or not. I want to share with you briefly about artificial sweeteners. According to the National Cancer Institute, numerous studies have been done on laboratory rats that have linked aspartame and saccharin to cancer. Aspartame is the worst; it's sold under the names NutraSweet and Equal. The second worst is saccharin, sold under the name Sweet'N Low. Please stop using these products! What makes aspartame so deadly to the body? Ten percent of aspartame is made up of methanol (wood alcohol), which is a deadly poison. Methanol breaks down into formic acid and formaldehyde in the body. Formaldehyde is a deadly neurotoxin known to destroy brain cells. An EPA assessment of methanol states that methanol "is considered a cumulative poison due to the low rate of excretion once it is absorbed. In the body, methanol is oxidized to formaldehyde and formic acid, both of these metabolites are toxic."

There are many forms of sugar, but I want to focus on three natural sweeteners that are less processed and create fewer fluctuations in blood-sugar levels. These sweeteners should be used in moderation. First is honey, one of oldest sweeteners. You should buy this locally from a farm. It has many beneficial properties especially if you have allergies. The second natural sweetener is maple syrup. Buy this locally as well, if you can. Make sure the label reads 100 percent pure, organic maple syrup. The third option is my favorite—coconut sugar. It's low on the glycemic index and high in nutrients and amino acids. Coconut sugar does not taste like coconut. It's an excellent choice for diabetics to use, as it will maintain the appropriate blood-sugar level.

The Aging Connection

At a cellular level, our skin is constantly being attacked by free radicals inside and outside of our body, and that creates inflammation.

Examples are sun, air, water, harsh soaps, skin- care products, internal disease, stress, lack of sleep, sugar consumption, and dehydration. At the top of the list is sugar and foods that rapidly convert into sugar, known as high-glycemic carbohydrates or "bad carbs." This free-radical theory makes it very easy to understand why we age. Free radicals are the start of acute and chronic disease; they are responsible for severe damage. Free radicals are simply troublemakers.

How free radicals are formed and the aging connection. Remember when you learned in school that our bodies are made up many different types of cells? Cells are composed of atoms and molecules. Each atom has one or more pairs of electrons. Electrons surround an atom in one or more shells. The innermost shell of the atom is full when it has two electrons. When the first shell is full, electrons begin to fill the second shell. When the second shell has eight electrons, it is full, and so on. The most important structural feature of an atom for determining its number of electrons in its outer shell. Because atoms seek to reach a state of maximum stability, an atom will try to fill it's outer shell by gaining or losing electrons. Atoms often will share its electrons by bonding together with other atoms in order to complete its outer shell. By sharing electrons, the atoms are bound together and satisfy the conditions of maximum stability for the molecules

When there is a weak bond, free radicals are formed. A free radical is a "bad" atom that is very unstable and trying to capture the needed electron to gain stability. Free radicals attack the nearest stable molecule, "stealing" its electron. When the "attacked" molecule loses its electron, it becomes a free radical itself, beginning a chain reaction. If the free-radical production becomes excessive, damage occurs in its path. Each time an electron pair is broken free radical damage accumulates and leads to aging.

Once we accept that our everyday lifestyle choices affect the way we age, we will be on our way to a healthier, longer life.

Nutrition is a major weapon against aging. What we eat fuels our body. Antioxidants in our food neutralize free radicals by giving one of their electrons, ending the damage. The antioxidants nutrients themselves do not become free radicals because they are very stable. Antioxidants prevent cell and tissue damage that could lead to cellular damage and disease There's that saying again, "We are what we eat."

I often wonder how it is possible that the majority of us deny our bodies and our brains the nutrients we need to fight aging. We have so much information and so many resources available to us. Why does this happen?

We must remember that failure to make a plan means planning to fail. We need to make the right nutritional decisions every day. When we realize how sugar triggers inflammation, and how the resulting chain reaction is ruining our health, we will find it easier to resist the package of chocolate cookies and the large bowl of pasta. We need to know that protein is essential to cellular repair. Protein supplies all of the essential amino acids needed for life. We need to shift the balance of what we are currently eating to good quality protein.

I would like to share with you about one of my sugar experiences. I was actually addicted to dark-chocolate-covered espresso beans. The product I was eating was full of refined sugar and highly addictive for me. I couldn't eat just two pieces; I needed to eat twenty. I bought *bags* of these treats and had them everywhere. I was definitely on the sugar-blues roller coaster. I knew I had to get off the roller coaster because my body just didn't feel right. I really didn't know how sick I was until later when I felt great and could compare the difference. I took a year of baby steps to kick the chocolate espresso bean addiction, and I have now totally switched to a healthy, organic dark chocolate. I still crave sugary chocolate, but I'm not putting all that processed sugar into my body anymore. I am able to satisfy my chocolate craving with just two squares of organic dark chocolate, and that's really all I need nutritionally. The best part is that dark chocolate is a superfood, the higher the cacao content the better. I have a piece or two of chocolate each day for the pleasure of eating chocolate, its nutritional value, and its calming effect.

You might wonder why trading one kind of chocolate for another is beneficial. There are definitely differences in chocolate. The cacao bean is the source of both cacao and cocoa powders. "Cacao" basically refers to the raw form of chocolate. The cacao bean is the base of any type of chocolate, unless it is an artifically flavored chocolate product. The actual cacao beans are found inside the fruit of the tree in fleshy, oval-shaped pods. The bean pods are harvested, fermented, and dried. When you see cacao nibs, powdered cacao, or cacao powder in the stores, the bean is in its raw state—uncooked, additive free, and unprocessed.

Cacao contains an abundance of antioxidants because it's raw and pure. It's also an amazing source of fiber, magnesium, essential fatty acids, iron, copper, zinc, sulfur, and calcium. It isn't until after the cacao beans are roasted and processed that they are called cocoa, but in the process the beans lose much of their nutritional benefits. There are two types of cocoa powder. The first type is Dutch-processed cocoa powder, which is made from cacao beans that have been washed with a potassium carbonate solution to alkalize pH and neutralize acidity. Dutch-processed cocoa is dark brown in color. The second type of cocoa is natural cocoa powder. It is reddish brown in color and is made from cocoa beans that are simply roasted and ground into a fine powder. Most cocoa powders have additives like sweeteners or cocoa butter.

The good, bad and basic material of life

When we eat a large volume of refined sugars or processed foods or a bowl of pasta, which converts to sugar in our bloodstream, the sugar triggers an insulin response from the pancreas to control the level of blood sugar in our body. Diabetics do not have a properly functioning pancreas; they suffer from high blood sugar, which must be treated with insulin shots. Diabetics with poorly controlled blood sugar actually age at a rate one-third faster than those who do not have diabetes. Constant high blood-sugar levels can cause kidney failure, blindness, heart attacks, and strokes.

You don't have to be diabetic to have an inflammatory response from sugar. Even a healthy body is damaged by sugar because of a process known as glycation. In this process foods rapidly convert to sugar in the bloodstream, in the same way that high-glycemic carbohydrates do. This has been shown to be detrimental to collagen, which can result in deep wrinkles. When glycation occurs in your skin, sugar molecules attach themselves to the collagen fibers. A gradual accumulation of irreversible chemical cross-links of collagen molecules is formed. This type of skin devastation causes the loss of skin elasticity. Healthy collagen strands normally slide over one another, which keeps skin elastic. The bond between sugar and collagen generates a large number of free radicals and lead to more inflammation. When glycation occurs the skin will become discolored and have deep lines and grooves over time. Besides the visible effects on our skin, glycation takes place in all parts of our body, destroying vital organs such as the kidneys, lungs, and brain.

Sugar causes inflammation in several ways. A diet high in pasta, cereals, bread, rice, potatoes, sweets, desserts, processed juices, and processed foods can actually lead to heart disease. When blood sugar goes up, it creates free radicals. Our cholesterol can also become oxidized, which means there's an environment within the cells where there is an excess of free radicals and a lack of antioxidants. Cholesterol can't dissolve in the blood. It must be transported through your bloodstream by carriers called lipoproteins, named because they're made of fat (lipids) and proteins. The two types of lipoproteins that carry cholesterol to and from cells are low-density lipoprotein, or LDL, and high-density lipoprotein, or HDL. Blood sugar increases insulin levels in the body, and then fats are stored. When too many fats are stored, obesity occurs. HDL cholesterol is considered "good" cholesterol because it helps remove LDL cholesterol from the arteries. Experts believe HDL acts as a scavenger, carrying LDL cholesterol away from the arteries and back to the liver, where it is broken down and passed from the body. HDL carries one-fourth to one-third of blood cholesterol. A healthy level of HDL cholesterol may also protect against heart attack and stroke, while low levels of HDL cholesterol have been shown to increase the risk of heart disease.

Here are some hidden sources of sugar in common foods.

A jar of regular pasta sauce contains about twelve grams of sugar (which is about three tablespoons) in a half-cup portion. (Most people use two or three times that amount.)

A six-ounce container of yogurt with fruit added typically has fourteen grams of sugar (more than three tablespoons) in that small container.

The sports drink Vitaminwater has thirty-one to thirty-two grams of sugar in each bottle. Coca-Cola, who manufactures Vitaminwater, was recently sued for deceptive labeling and marketing of the product. Coca-Cola's defense lawyer argued in court that "no consumer could reasonably be misled into thinking Vitaminwater was a healthy beverage."

Our Standard American Diet (SAD) focus is on meat, potatoes, dairy products, and refined and processed carbohydrates. And our sugar addiction has made the United States the leaders in cancer, stroke, and heart problems. We as Americans are the most overweight nation on the globe.

How do we regulate the amount of sugar we eat? The glycemic index (GI) can help. It is one of the keys to looking and feeling younger. The glycemic index is a number associated with a particular type of food that indicates the food's effect on a person's blood glucose (also called blood sugar) level. The GI represents the total rise in a person's blood-sugar level following consumption of the food, although it may not represent how quickly the blood sugar rises. The steepness of the rise can be influenced by a number of other factors, such as the quantity of fat eaten with the food. The GI is useful for understanding how the body breaks down carbohydrates and only takes into account the available carbohydrates (total carbohydrate minus fiber) in a food. Although the food may contain fats and other components that contribute to the total rise in blood sugar, these effects are not reflected in the GI.

Carbohydrates—Complex carbohydrates have a" bad" influence on blood sugar. They include corn, pasta, rice, and bread. These foods can trigger a rapid increase in blood sugar, which prevents us from being able to burn or utilize our body fat for energy, so it gets stored. To stay young looking, we need to have a slow, steady release of insulin into our bloodstream. "Good" low-glycemic carbohydrates are packed with vitamins, minerals, and antioxidants and can be eaten fresh or frozen. They slow aging while supplying essential energy. These carbohydrates also contain water, which hydrates the skin and body. Low-glycemic carbohydrates include spinach, blueberries, shrimp, and turkey.

Proteins—Proteins are the basic material of life, so the body can't grow or function without them. The human body manufactures only twelve of the twenty-two amino acids that are essential for life. The remaining ten must be provided through the foods we eat. However, the SAD rarely contains enough protein to maintain and repair cell and skin health. Protein is essential to cellular repair. The building blocks of our cells are amino acids, which are also used by the cells to repair themselves. Without adequate protein our bodies enter an accelerated aging mode. The US Department of Agriculture recommends women eat at least sixty-five to seventy grams of protein daily. Men need at least seventy-five to eighty grams. Great sources of protein are quinoa, fish, skinless chicken and turkey, seafood, and egg whites. A single serving of grilled chicken breast has twenty-eight grams of protein. Half a cup of navy beans has seven grams of protein.

We can't store protein in our bodies. If you want to keep your face and body firm and toned, you need to eat a fresh supply of high-quality protein every day—three meals and two snacks.

If you don't like fish, try flaxseed oil or ground flaxseeds in smoothies or on your salad to get omega-3 fatty acids and protein.

Fats—Fats can be incorporated into the cell membrane for good or for bad. Chemically, fats and oils are made up of chains of carbon molecules edged with hydrogen and oxygen molecules. When the carbon chain is completely full of hydrogen, it's called saturated fat (like butter and lard). When the chains are missing two hydrogen molecules, it's called a monounsaturated fat (like olive oil). If a carbon chain is missing four or more hydrogen molecules, this type of fat is called polyunsaturated (like corn oil and fish oil—omega 3s). Mono- and polyunsaturated fats are liquid at room temperature. Each type of fat has different properties and has different effects on the body.

Karen Mayo
Certified Nutrition Health and Lifestyle Coach

"Good" Foods Low-Gylcemic		"Bad" Foods High-Glycemic	
Water	Apple	Acorn Squash	Cereal
Oatmeal	Grapes	Baked Beans	Cornstarch
Eggs	Plum	Beets	Croissant
Protein Powder	Shrimp	Black-eyed Peas	Croutons
Peanut Butter	Mayonnaise	Butternut Squash	Doughnut
Tahini	Plain Yogurt	Cooked Carrots	English Muffin
Olives	Deli Meat	Corn	Granola
Beef	Ham	French Fries	Grits
Cheese	Soy Milk	Hubbard Squash	Melba Toast
Salsa	Spirulina	Lima Beans	Muffin
Black Beans	Tempeh	Parsnips	Noodles
Kidney Beans	Egg Substitute	Peas	Instant Oatmeal
Ground Turkey	Oil	Pinto Beans	Pancake
Soy Sausage	Peanuts	Potato	Popcorn
Chicken	Swordfish	Refried Beans	Rice
Turkey Susage	Peanuts	Sweet Potato	Rolls
Salmon	Swordfish	Turnip	Taco Shell
Turkey	Tuna Steak	Banana	Tortilla
Canned Tuna	Tomato Sauce	Cranberries	Udon Noodles
Canned Chicken	Spinich	Dates	Waffle
Soy Burgers	Carrots	Fig	BBQ Sauce
Cottage Cheese	Orange	Guava	Ketchup
Almonds	Pear	Mango	Cocktail Sauce
Macadamia Nuts	Pinapple	Papaya	Honey
Avocado	Brussels Sprouts	Prunes	Jelly
Tofu	Eggplant	Raisins	Sugar
Tomato	Sauerkraut	Fruit Juice	Maple Syrup
Lettuce	Hot Dogs	Vegetable Juice	Teriyaki Sauce
Onion	Chickpeas	Bagel	Chocolate
Mushrooms	Lamb	Biscuit	Corn Chips
Cucumber	Pork	Bread Crumbs	Ice Cream
Blueberries	Dill Pickles	Bread	Potato Chips
Milk	Soy Beans	Steak Sauce	Pretzels
Broccoli	Asparagus	Bulger	Saltine Crackers
Zucchini	Peach	Sweet Relish	Molasses

WHAT CAUSES CRAVINGS?

*T*he body is wonderful; it never makes mistakes. It knows when to wake up, when to go to the bathroom, and when to go to sleep. Your lungs are always breathing, and the heart never misses a beat. The body repairs itself when you get hurt, and the body knows to maintain a temperature of 98.6 degrees. The amazing childbirth process goes to show that the body is perfect.

When it comes to food cravings, it's the behaviors in your lifestyle that are causing these cravings. Don't view cravings as a weakness, because these impulses are the body's way of telling you there's something missing from your plate. Deconstruct those cravings by using the following list.

Causes of Cravings

1. Dehydration can trick your body into thinking it's hungry, but really all you need to do is to drink a full glass of water and wait twenty minutes.

2. Emotional eating is caused when you are dissatisfied with a relationship, bored, stressed out, uninspired, or lack enough

exercise. Lack of a spiritual connection can also cause emotional eating.

3. Seasonal cravings are really to tell us what foods to eat. In spring we crave more greens. In the summer, people usually crave food like salads, fruits, and ice cream, which are cooling foods. Fall is usually the time we crave earthy vegetables like apples, pumpkin, nuts, and squashes. In the winter we usually crave soups and stews and holiday foods as well.

4. A lack of vitamins and nutrients will create very strange cravings.

5. Hormonal changes in women will make us crave foods that normally we would not eat.

When these cravings come up, recognize them, and use the chart to see how you can eat healthier given the situation.

Karen Mayo

Certified Nutrition Health and Lifestyle Coach

If you crave this...	What you really need is...	And here are the healthy foods that have it:
Chocolate	Magnesium	Raw nuts and seeds, legumes, fruits
Sweets	Chromium	Broccoli, grapes, cheese, dried beans, calves liver, chicken
	Carbon	Fresh fruits
	Phosphorus	Chicken, beef, liver, poultry, fish, eggs, dairy, nuts, legumes, grains
	Sulfur	Cranberries, horseradish, cruciferous vegetables, kale, cabbage
	Tryptophan	Cheese, liver, lamb, raisins, sweet potato, spinach
Bread, toast	Nitrogen	High protein foods: fish, meat, nuts, beans
Oily snacks, fatty foods	Calcium	Mustard and turnip greens, broccoli, kale, legumes, cheese, sesame
Coffee or tea	Phosphorous	Chicken, beef, liver, poultry, fish, eggs, dairy, nuts, legumes
	Sulfur	Egg yolks, red peppers, muscle protein, garlic, onion, cursiferous vegetables
	NaCl (salt)	Sea salt, apple cider vinegar (on salad)
	Iron	Meat, fish and poultry, seaweed, greens, black cherries
Alcohol, recreational drugs	Protein	Meat, poultry, seafood, dairy, nuts
	Avenin	Granola, oatmeal
	Calcium	Mustard and turnip greens, broccoli, kale, legumes, cheese, sesame
	Glutamine	Supplement glutamine powder for withdrawal, raw cabbage juice
	Potassium	Sun-dried black olives, potato peel broth, seaweek, bitter greens
Chewing ice	Iron	Meat, fish, poultry, seaweed, greens, black cherries
Burned food	Carbon	Fresh fruits
Soda and other carbonated drinks	Calcium	Mustard and turnip greens, broccoli, kale, legumes, cheese, sesame
Salty foods	Cloride	Raw goat milk, fish, unrefined sea salt
Acid foods	Magnesium	Raw nuts and seeds, legumes, fruits
Preference for liquids rather than solids	Water	Flavor water with lemon or lime. You need 8 to 10 glasses per day.
Preference for solids rather than liquids	Water	You have been so dehydrated for so long that you have lost your thirst. Flavor water with lemon or lime. You need 8 to 10 glasses.
Cook drinks	Manganese	Walnuts, almonds, pecans, pineapple, blueberries
Pre-menstrual cravings	Zinc	Red meats (especially organ meats), seafood, leafy vegetables, root vegetables
General overeating	Silicon	Nuts, seeds; avoid refined starches
	Tryptophan	Cheese, liver, lamb, raisins, sweet potato, spinach
	Tyrosine	Vitamin c supplements or orange, green, red fruits and vegetables
Lack of appetite	Vitamin B1	Nuts, seeds, beans, liver and other organ meats
	Vitamin B3	Tuna, halibut, beef, chicken, turkey, pork, seeds and legumes
	Manganese	Walnuts, almonds, pecans, pineapple, blueberries
	Chloride	Raw goat milk, fish, unrefined sea salt
Tobacco	Silicon	Nuts, seeds; avoid refined starches
	Tyrosine	Vitamin c supplements or orange, green and red fruits and vegetables

CHAPTER FOUR

THE RAW DIFFERENCES

*I*n the late 1800s, people in Europe were juicing cabbage, potatoes, and beetroot to treat ulcers, cancer, and leukemia. By the time you're finished reading these few sentences, four Americans have had a heart attack., Another four have had a stroke or heart failure. Heart attack is a leading cause of death worldwide. Cancer kills 7.6 million people annually. Deaths from cancer are projected to reach over 11 million annually by 2030.

Throughout the world, 171 million people have been diagnosed with diabetes, and over 500 million people are clinically obese. World Health Organization states that obesity is one of the most serious public health problems of the twenty-first century.

Why are we so sick?

Check out the USDA food pyramid from 1992. The Standard American Diet (SAD) has us eating six to eleven servings of bread, cereal, rice, and pasta a day.

The majority of diseases and chronic illness conditions can be directly attributed to the consumption of too many processed foods that are high in sugar and salt, which seriously increase our risk of cancer, diabetes, and heart disease.

Every cell in our body has a lifespan. New cells are constantly replacing dead cells. Over the next seven years, every single cell in our bodies will regenerate. This amazing cell-replacement process is very delicate and complete, but it is not perfect. The new cells may contain errors; this is how we age. The errors in our cells increase with the amount of free radicals we take in every day. Examples of toxic free radicals are smoking, second hand smoke, drinking alcohol, and eating unhealthy, processed foods with added sugar and salt. All of these things speed up the aging process and develop disease.

Juicing has no Pulp.

Fruits, vegetables, and plant-based foods contain natural antioxidants that neutralize harmful free radicals and protect our cells from further damage.

Has anyone juiced as part of a healthy lifestyle? Even if you haven't, you've probably seen juice bars, smoothie cafes, or an elixir café. These establishments are popping up everywhere around the United States. Do you think this is a new trend? Actually, juicing has been around since the late 1800s, as a health practice

Juicing makes it easier to consume the recommended daily servings of eight fruits and vegetables, which serve a major role in ensuring a healthy lifestyle. One large glass of pure, raw, fresh juice per day will increase energy, strengthen your bones, clear your skin, lower your risk of disease, and improve your immune system. Try juicing a wide variety of fruits, vegetables, and herbs.

Be sure that you don't completely replace whole fruits and vegetables with juicing. The fiber in the fruits and vegetables are very important for eliminating toxins and preventing chronic illness. Incorporate juices into a well-balanced, high-fiber, whole-food, healthy lifestyle.

The juices should taste delightful. When you begin to juice, you will notice that the taste of fresh, raw juice is strong and different. Once you change your eating lifestyle to a whole-food way of eating, you will notice that both the juice and the pulp from fresh juice offer pure bursts of true flavor.

When you are just beginning to juice, try using three mild ingredients, like apples or carrots, to one strong ingredient, like cabbage, broccoli, or dark, leafy-green vegetables. Start acclimating to juices by drinking one glass a day for several days to allow your body to adjust. Work your way up to as many as two glasses a day.

Juice Machines—Two Basic Types

Masticating—This juice machine squeezes fruits and vegetables through gears that crush and force the produce through a fine stainless-steel strainer. The pulp is continuously extracted. This process extracts more nutrients, generates less heat and friction, and preserves more enzymes.

Centrifugal—This type of juicer uses a spinning basket that shreds the fruits and vegetables then forces the juice through a fine stainless-steel strainer. This type of juicer causes oxidation of nutrients by the air that comes into the juice.

Choosing a Juice Machine

Ease of Use—If a machine is easy to use and easy clean up, you will use it more often. The goal of the juicer is to extract the most juice from the fruit or vegetable as possible. Juicers that eject the pulp outside the machine yield less juice then those that keep the pulp in the basket.

Reliability—Look for a five- to-ten-year warranty on the juicer's motor and parts. Look for a company that supplies replacement parts for the juicer at a reasonable cost.

Benefits of Juicing

Easy Assimilation—Once freed from the cellulose, the juice can be absorbed into the cells of the body within fifteen minutes, compared to the hour or more with it is still in the pulp. The juice contains vitamins A, C, and E, enzymes, and important minerals like iron, copper, potassium, iodine, and magnesium. I also can't forget to mention the phytochemicals, which are antioxidants. These compounds occur naturally in blueberries and garlic.

Water Supply—Juicing is a quick way to supply our cells with nutrients. Our cells consist mostly of water, which is essential for proper function. Raw juice supplies the water needed to replenish lost fluids. Raw juicing provides all the necessary vitamins, minerals, and enzymes that promote the alkalinity of body fluids, which is vital for metabolic function and proper immune function.

Cleansing Action—When the fiber is removed, raw fruit juice has a laxative effect, which helps rid the body of toxins. Chlorophyll, found only in plants, enhances the body's ability to produce hemoglobin, which enhances the delivery of oxygen to the cells.

Detoxifying your body's systems by cleansing your digestive track and colon will help clear your mind and balance your moods. Your metabolism will become more efficient, and if you follow the whole-food lifestyle, your body will revert to its natural weight.

Smoothies have Pulp

What does a healthy whole-food plate look like? It should offer proteins, carbohydrates, fat, vitamins, minerals, enzymes, phytochemicals—which are antioxidants—fiber, and water to promote the growth of beautiful, new, vibrant cells.

We are all in busy land, and we often don't take the time to eat healthy or chew properly, which makes our digestive system work harder to get nutrients. Over time the stressed digestive system enzymes and our weakened stomach acids can't break down the food enough to utilize the nutritional value in the foods. When our bodies fail to absorb these nutrients day after day, week after week, year after year, we become weak and more susceptible to sickness and chronic disease.

Eat food in its whole, natural state. When we properly chew fresh fruits and vegetables, we get all the benefits of the pulp, which is their amazing flesh, along with its vitamins, minerals, enzymes, and antioxidants. If we don't chew properly, all the goodness gets trapped because we haven't released the components of the food. Digestion begins in your mouth, as soon as you start to chew your food; digestive enzymes found in the saliva begin to break down the food in your mouth. It's important to chew your food thoroughly to achieve maximum absorption of all your vitamins and minerals. To get into the habit of chewing foods thoroughly, try counting your chews and aiming for thirty to forty per bite.

Benefits of Smoothies

Unlike juicing, the product you get from pulping is full of fiber. It takes longer to digest the pulp of fruits and vegetables, which increases the absorption of nutrients. Pulping helps eliminate toxins, lower cholesterol, lower the risk of heart disease, prevent varicose veins and constipation, and helps to prevent chronic illness.

You are satisfied longer when you drink pulp. The body is also nourished longer, and the fiber gives the sense of satisfaction when you pulp fruits and vegetables with herbs, nuts, seeds, and whole grains.

Smoothie Machines

You may want a blender, Vitamix, or food processor in addition to a juice machine, since there are some fruits like a banana and vegetables like an avocado that don't juice well. Some ingredients, such as flaxseeds, dry herbs, and wheat germ are easier to add to blended drinks than to juices. Blenders are better at pulping than food processors. Most blended drinks or smoothies call for some juice. It's best if fresh raw fruits and vegetables are first juiced using a juice extractor, than added to a pulping machine to complete the recipe.

Juicing and smoothies both have their place in living a healthy lifestyle

Notes:

Fruits supply the body with natural sugar called fructose, which it uses for fuel. The natural sugar makes the vegetable juices more enjoyable to drink. The fiber of fresh, raw fruit is an important food to eat whole as well.

Diabetics and people prone to yeast infections and hypoglycemia need to watch how much fruit they eat because of the rapid rise in blood sugar that they cause. Fruit juices should be drunk in the morning to lunch hours, and vegetables juice should be drunk from lunch into the evening.

Ready to use juices, like canned or bottled juices, are processed at high heat and may contain added ingredients such as sugar, artificial flavorings, stabilizers, thickeners, thinners, and chemical preservatives. Should you choose this type of juice, look for pure juice with no sugar or additives.

Buy fresh fruits, vegetables, and herbs for your juicer, and plan to use them within a day or two. Longer storage will destroy the live enzymes in the plants. Store produce covered, in the refrigerator.

A handy rule of thumb to remember is that one pound of produce yields one to one and one-half cups of fresh juice.

Use fresh herbs for juicing if they are available. Organic, dried herbs can be bought at a farm or health-food store.

All fruits, vegetables, and herbs (even organic) should be washed, scrubbed, and soaked in a tub of cool water, with two parts white vinegar to three parts water. This will remove any soil and bacteria that the produce may have picked up during transportation and handling.

Choosing organic will hugely decrease the load on your body's elimination system since you won't have to deal with a host of chemical fertilizers, pesticides, and fungicides.

Healthy amounts of juicing complete our daily requirement for fresh fruits and vegetables. Most importantly, juicing is the very best way to obtain the nutrients and phytochemical those foods are meant to provide for our health.

Use the pulp, which contains a lot of fiber and nutrients, for frozen desserts, soups, sauces, vegetable stocks, dressings, or baked goods.

Cleansing and Detoxing and Fasting Oh My!

Modern science is pointing to the fact that in today's stressful and toxic environment, it's more important now than ever to have a whole-food lifestyle and a safe cleansing program for your body.

The goal of cleansing, detoxing, or fasting is to release and eliminate toxins stored in the colon and in fat cells of the body. Short-term cleanses or juice fasts work best with a whole-food lifestyle, regular exercise, and a strong commitment to inner growth and spiritual development.

If we detox/cleanse a little bit every day, we reduce the risk of toxic buildup in our body's system of elimination. Make small changes every day to decrease the toxic load on your organs.

Fasting

You probably haven't thought of it as fasting, but you are already fasting between the time you go to sleep at night and when you wake up in the morning—hence the name break-fast. Get it! That's why breakfast is such an important meal. Make sure your first meal after your nightly fast is healthy!

What's the most important meal of the day? As I mentioned previously, we have been told for years to, always eat a good breakfast. That's because you are breaking the fast that you experience each night when you sleep. Drinking a warm cup of water first thing in the morning with lemon squeezed is the best morning routine. The acid from the lemon helps clean out the digestive tract and acts like a detergent to break down stored fats. Remember too that lemon has a very alkalizing effect on the body after it is consumed.

Fasting Choices

There are many fasting choices that you can learn about. Here is one that I recommend.

The lemonade fast is, a powerful fast for the kidneys, digestive system, and liver. Lemon and lime are rich sources of vitamins and minerals, and they help to reduce accumulation of toxins in the liver and stomach. Lemon also fights infections and builds up immunity. One hundred percent pure maple syrup supplies vitamins and minerals and enough sugar to sustain energy and curbs sweet cravings. Cayenne pepper works as a stimulant to break up mucus and to provide warmth to the digestive system. Ground ginger works together with the cayenne pepper to speed up metabolism, burn fat faster, and boost circulation. Here is the recipe. Combine eight cups pure water, the juice of four fresh lemons or limes, three Tablespoons pure maple syrup, one-eighth teaspoon of cayenne pepper, and a pinch of ground ginger. Combine and drink six to twelve cups per day at room temperature. Make fresh daily.

What Is Detox, and Who Needs It?

Detox is a cleansing program to boost vitality and to boost your immune system. During the detox process, cells begin to recover from the stress that leads to inflammation. Cells also extract nutrients from the greens consumed, and these nutrients restore natural balance and function.

Tidbit about Toxins

The body will use beneficial food, air, and water, to promote health and vitality, and it will eliminate the toxins that we take in. When the body doesn't eliminate the toxins through the natural process of sweat, urine, and natural bowel function, the toxins accumulate, and the body will become toxic. Your body already produces toxins as a by-product of your metabolism, stress, and exercise. Modern life exposes you to thousands of toxins every day, including the chemicals found in many highly processed foods.

Toxins can be found in exhaust fumes, secondhand smoke, insecticides, pesticides, herbicides, food preservatives, food colorings, food flavorings, food thickeners, food enhancers, and chemical and industrial pollution.

How Do Toxins Cause Damage?

Toxins are often stored in fat and other tissues in the body, and they build up over time. Our bodies are supposed to be capable of eliminating what we don't need, but the sheer quantity of toxins we are now exposed to forces our liver and kidneys to work overtime. This increases our risk for chronic illness and disease.

The most significant damage happens at the cellular level. Let's go back to the basics of all matter, known as an atom. An atom consists of the nucleus, comprised of protons and neutrons, surrounded by electrons. As we have learned, an atom that has lost an electron is known as a free radical. Free radicals never stop in their quest to steal an electron to complete themselves. This process decreases the body's natural chemicals, disrupts internal biochemistry, and creates dis-ease in the body.

Toxins and Hormone Imbalance

There are insecticides and pesticides that mimic the action of our own hormones. Hormones run essential body functions, like human reproduction, energy production, and blood-sugar management. Toxic chemicals are so close to our natural hormones in structure that they create hormone imbalances. This leads to problems with the management of many essential body processes.

Are We Healthy?

Over the past few decades, the United States has become the most overfed nation in the world, yet we are an undernourished nation.

When we feel sick, where do we go? We often hurry straight to the doctor's office looking for a quick fix. We get pills for feeling sad (the happy pill). We get pills for feeling anxious (the chill pill). We get pills for sniffles (the Z-Pac or other antibiotics). We get pills for erectile dysfunction (the blue pill). We get pills for high blood pressure, indigestion, high cholesterol; you get the picture. There's a pill for anything that's ailing us. Yet the National Institutes of Health website says that "even with the large variety of medications available, current middle-aged Americans report feeling less healthythan the generation before them."

The leading causes of death in the United States are, in order of most to least deaths, heart disease, cancer, chronic lower-respiratory disease (which includes chronic bronchitis—inflammation of the bronchi; emphysema—air sacs are damaged; asthma—spasms in the bronchi; smoking, and inhalants), stroke, accidents, Alzheimer's disease, diabetes, influenza and pneumonia, and kidney disease.

Why are we less healthy as a population, in spite of all the incredible medical advancements in the past fifty years,? Even our pets are overweight and unhealthy. Do you think it could be we are avoiding responsibility for own health and the health of our families? Are we relying on prescription medication, which often treats the symptoms but does not treat our actual health problem?

How Do We Eliminate the Toxins?

What are the major routes of elimination in your body? The major organs of elimination are the lungs, liver, bowels, skin, and kidneys. Mother Nature has supplied our bodies with a variety of effective routes for getting rid of toxins. However, most of us the elimination pathways are on permanent overload and under a great deal of strain. The lungs have to deal with secondhand smoke, airborne pollution, lack of fresh air, and no exercise. The liver is overtaxed trying to filter the blood and deal with our fatty diets, manmade chemicals, alcohol consumption, and the vast array of prescription and recreational drugs. Our bowels are often accumulating waste, instead of eliminating it. Our skin, which is the largest organ of the human body, is not being regularly exfoliated. Our kidneys, which are the blood cleaners, are often starved of water they need to flush out toxins. Kidneys receive filtered blood from the body and filter it back again into the bloodstream. Be good to those poor kidneys, and drink more water.

There's one more very important system that is affected by an overload of toxins, too much stress, busy schedules, late nights, not sleeping properly, and the stress of whatever else life throws at you. It's the major system in your body that governs and controls the organs of the elimination system—the nervous system. And it's just plain and simply exhausted. When the nervous system is exhausted, it's not doing its job. A tired you is a toxic you.

Switching to Pure Whole Foods

Detoxing is about giving your body a rest from the hustle and bustle of life, and that begins by cleaning up your plate. The idea here is to reduce the amount of filtering your liver and kidneys have to do before you can begin the process of assimilating and digesting the nutrients. When these organs are functioning well, you will get more out of your food and have more energy. Your overall energy levels will improve, your health will improve, and you will begin to lose weight. Whole foods are rich in two crucial detox nutrients. Antioxidants zip through the body cleaning up the disease-causing free radicals. Fiber is the second crucial detox nutrient, which helps to ensure that you move your bowels every day so toxins are not reabsorbed back into your body, making the toxic overload worse. If we make small changes every day to decrease the toxic overload on the organs, we will create a lasting change. It just takes a little bit every day to reduce the risk of toxic buildup in our bodies.

There are lots of ways to detox, from a weekend plan to a lifestyle change. It starts with you and your short- and long-term goals. As I mentioned earlier, choosing organic is better for some fruits and veg-etables like celery, apples, strawberries, peaches, spinach, nectarines, grapes, sweet bell peppers, potatoes, blueberries, lettuce, kale, and collard greens. This list of produce is known as the dirty dozen or the twelve items that are most contaminated with chemicals. If you can't swing buying organic, remember to wash all your fruits and vegetables thoroughly in the vinegar wash I described previously. Washing will decrease the excessive amount of chemical load that your body's filtration system has to eliminate.

As a reminder, the clean fifteen, or the produce that is least contaminated with chemicals, are onions, corn, pineapple, avocado, sweet peas, mangoes, eggplant, cantaloupe, kiwi, cabbage, watermelon, sweet potatoes, grapefruit, and mushrooms.

Best Foods for Detoxing

Beets and beet greens are known for cleansing properties. Beets are loaded with powerful antioxidants that help detox the liver and kidneys.

Celery is loaded with antioxidants, an excellent detoxifying ingredient. It has amazing diuretic properties and is especially beneficial to the kidneys. Celery lowers uric-acid levels in the blood, which reduces the risk of developing kidney stones. Celery is delicious when it is blended with a cored apple and lemon juice.

Artichokes, like celery, lower uric-acid levels. They also contain compounds that assist in the production and elimination of bile, which is the fluid discharge of toxins that the liver produces. This process helps to ensure that toxins are efficiently condensed and removed from the body.

Apples are loaded with powerful antioxidants that may prevent the growth of cancer cells in the bowel and liver.

Greens are full of chlorophyll. They help the liver rid the body of harmful environmental and dietary toxins like pesticides, herbicides, and heavy metals. Spinach, kale, alfalfa, spirulina, chlorella, arugula, collard greens, Swiss chard, wheat grass, and blue-green algae are great examples of delicious greens.

Garlic is a pungent bulb that helps to support the liver. Garlic can be eaten raw or cooked. Garlic contains many more healthful components such as selenium-a mineral that increases the action of antioxidants, which assists the liver in detoxification. Arginine—an amino acid important for relaxing the blood vessels, which eases blood pressure in the liver. Vitamin B6—helps lower homocysteine levels in the body, thus acting as an anti-inflammatory substance which inhibits inflammation in the liver. Vitamin C—the body's primary antioxidant defender protecting against cellular oxidation; a major contributor to liver cell damage.

Asparagus, broccoli, cauliflower, cabbage, carrots, turmeric and oregano are full of sulfur and glutathione. These foods help in the detoxification process, especially when eaten raw.

Citrus fruit such as lemons, limes, kiwis, and oranges are rich in vitamin C. These foods transform harmful toxins into digestible material and support the liver in the cleansing process. Kiwi is a super fruit that is loaded with more vitamin C than oranges.

Benefits of Detox/Cleansing

You will have a leaner and cleaner *you*! You will reduce your intake of toxins, and the toxic load on your organs will decrease, giving your body a chance to clean up and feel great. You will notice an increase in energy, fewer aches and pains, better sleep patterns, and see improvement in skin tone and texture. To be successful at this cleanse, you may want to clean house! Look through your cupboards and on your countertops and get rid of all the processed food, animal protein, gluten products, caffeine, alcohol, and sugars. Add in more whole, gluten-free grains, low-sugar fruits, herbal tea, lots of vegetables, protein supplements, and drink more water.

Successful Ways to Detox/Cleanse and Eliminate Toxins

1) Clean house by purging your cabinets, cupboards, and countertops.
2) Use the buddy system, and ask a friend to join you.
3) Ease into the detox; take baby steps toward a start date.
4) Massage is a great way to cleanse your body. Massage simulates the lymphatic system, which may boost the immune system. Massage also increases circulation.
5) Do the being grateful exercise. Write down all the things for which you are grateful.
6) Meditate or spend time just being quiet for thirty minutes before bed.
7) Take warm baths with salts.
8) Consume mindfully; know where your food comes from.
9) Drink warm lemon water upon arising in the morning. To promote proper elimination, drink fruit juices in the morning and at lunch. Drink vegetable juices from mid-afternoon into the evening.
10) Drink organ- supporting herbal teas (detox teas). Tea blend of organic burdock root, stinging nettle leaf, ginger root, dandelion root are all great ways to promote a healthy cleanse of the two primary filtering organs, the liver and kidneys.
11) Exercise, sweating is the body's primary way of releasing toxins and waste.
12) Enjoy sauna's or baths along with dry brushing your skin, which stimulates circulation before you get into the shower. You will need a natural bristle brush, bath mitts, or loofah, When brushing your skin, use light pressure and a continuous circular motion and always towards the heart. Cover your entire skin *except* the breasts on women.
13) Add phylum seeds to your drinking water, and drink a minimum of ten glasses of pure, filtered water a day.

CHAPTER FIVE

PREPARE FOR THE MINDFUL EATING MENU PLAN

This step-by-step program will supercharge your health by clearing your body of impurities. You have the plan in your hand to build new health habits that will result in some surprising benefits, including looking younger, increased energy, and better sleep. Making small changes will help you transition to a sustainable, long-lasting, healthy lifestyle.

Let's begin by taking a little time to fill out the health questionnaire in the handbook. Make a note of the symptoms that you have now or have experienced in the past three months. At the end of the program, we will revisit this questionnaire so you can see how your symptoms have lessened or disappeared. The handbook journal is a way to set your goals for better health and to keep you on track for success. Journal pages provide space for you to write down your thoughts and emotions on a weekly and daily basis.

"Journaling or expressive writing is a simple, gentle, and inexpensive healing technique. I consider it a powerful therapeutic tool to learn more about yourself and become aware of how your mind and emotions can influence you physically."—Dr. Andrew Weil

There are three phases of the plan: the preparation, the transition, and the new, healthy version of you.

Phase One—Prepare to Cleanse Your Bloodstream

Phase one is designed to relax the body's organs and to allow them to release old toxins, excess fat, and extra water. This phase is designed to give you some time to make small changes each day, building on the previous day.

During weeks one and two, you will be crowding out certain acid-forming or stress foods and adding in more easily digested or more alkaline foods. A change in anything you do is not easy, especially eating, but there is comfort in knowing that what you will be eating in the next month will save your life. The mind can and will produce a million excuses why you don't have to change your life. Listen to the excuses your mind gives you. Write them down, and when you read them, you will realize they are only excuses—nothing more. Developing new, healthy habits is going to take time. You should also make a list of *why* you are creating new, healthy habits, so when your mind is giving you excuses, you can silence it.

There are six types of foods that you will skip during this program. The first is processed or packaged foods and beverages. Let your body rest a bit, and enjoy foods in their purest form.

The second food to skip is added sugar, artificial sweeteners, and fructose. As we have discussed, these are highly addictive and suppress the immune system. Honey or coconut sugar is all right in small amounts.

The third food group to skip is all dairy. Heartburn, digestive upset, diarrhea, and chronic ear and sinus infections are all linked to this common allergen. Even if you are not allergic, your body can benefit from a dairy break. Transition over to unsweetened almond milk, hemp milk, coconut milk, or hazelnut milk. Instead of eating cheese, you can have a handful of almonds.

The fourth food to skip is gluten. This wheat protein is difficult for many people to digest. If you sometimes feel bloated, fatigued, or moody, you may be gluten intolerant and not even know it. A good transition food is brown rice or quinoa.

The fifth item to skip is caffeinated teas, coffee, or caffeine; these are false energy boosters that can mask lack of sleep or bad food choices. Offset headaches by switching to de-café black or green tea. I know this one is always a tough one. Go slowly, and tell yourself that you're just taking a break or experimenting. Try cutting your caffeine intake in half for this first week of transition; you may want to try decaffeinated tea or coffee. Try a warm cup of water with lemon squeezed in it; this will really get you moving in the morning.

The sixth item to skip is alcohol. It can mess with your metabolism and interfere with sleep, and it also makes your liver work overtime.

During week one we will be going back to the basics with simple meals made from only purifying fruits and vegetables that power both body and mind. This will allow the vital organs and digestive system to focus on cleansing itself. Taking a break from processed foods and common allergens puts you more in touch with your body and gives your kidneys and liver a break. You may experience a headache, head cold, or fatigue; it's your body healing and working to get rid of the toxins. Hang in there! By the end of week you will feel lighter. You will be more energized, and you will definitely be thinking more clearly and be motivated for week two.

Remember to drink lots of water, and flavor it with a squeeze of lemon or lime.

Your mindful movement for the week is to choose an exercise you love, and have fun doing it for thirty minutes for three days. Turn up the music, and shake your groove thang baby! In addition to your thirty minutes of exercise, take the stairs instead of the elevator. Park your car farther away in the parking lot from the front door of the store. Be careful your first week, though. You don't want to break something.

The affirmation of the week is about you, the physical human being. Repeat "I am fearless" at all times of the day. Write it in the journal, and say it to yourself in the mirror. This statement is great when your mind is giving you excuses that will self-sabotage your efforts.

The mindful meditation of the week is to be mindful about your relationship with your food. Visualize the care and love with which the food was prepared. Think about how it felt going into your mouth, the textures, and how you enjoyed each nutritious bite.

Write in your journal each night before bed, or journal in the morning. You will want to go to bed earlier during this program. Give your body more rest and the healing it needs. Each weekend, journal about your greatest accomplishment for the week, biggest challenge you had that week, and what your main health concern was for that week. Did you experience self-sabotage? If so, how did you silence your mind?

In week two, with all the excited energy and renewed sense of self, you should no longer be experiencing withdrawal symptoms. This week you should really be feeling the benefits of eating more nutrient-rich whole foods. You should have increased awareness of how your body is reacting to the foods you are eating. If you're experiencing cravings, they should decrease by the end of this week. You should be sleeping much better and feeling happier than you have in a while.

The movement of the week is to do thirty minutes of exercise for five days, add in stretching for ten minutes before and after you exercise. Turn on the music, get up, and dance!

The affirmation for this week is about the relationships in your life. Fill in the blank in the sentence, "I am grateful for_____," and know the reason why. Being grateful is a very positive vibration, and it makes you feel good too. Repeat the affirmation from last week. You now have two affirmations to use every day. Repeat as necessary. You can repeat the grateful affirmation every day this week if you like; you may have many reasons to be grateful.

The mindful meditation of the week is to be mindful of your breathing while you are sitting cross-legged on a cushion or on a chair with your eyes closed and your back straight. You may focus your attention on the movement of your abdomen when breathing in and out, or on the awareness of the breath as it goes in and out the nostrils. Put your right hand on your heart and left hand on your abdomen. The point isn't to clear your thoughts; it's to be aware of your thoughts and learn to let them be. As thoughts come up, return to focusing on the object of meditation, in this case the breathing. Close your eyes, and deeply breathe to fill your abdomen all the way. Hold for a count of four, and slowly breathe out for a count of four. Do this four times. Open your eyes slowly, and you should have a different aspect on things.

You will continue your journal writing in the morning or evening. Write your affirmations of the week and your reasons why. Each weekend journal about your greatest accomplishment for the week, your biggest challenge, what your main health concerns were, if you experienced self-sabotage, and, if so, how you silenced your mind.

Phase Two—The Transition

Now you are ready to enter phase two. You have learned how to eat clean, and now you feel amazing. It's crucial during these last few weeks to stick to the program. Your body is in the middle of a cleansing process. It's time to fine-tune your newly developed mindful eating habits. If you have eaten (or are eating) any of the stress-causing foods or acidic-forming foods, you will need to repeat phase one before moving on to phase two.

Weeks three and four are about living a healthy lifestyle and having a balanced pH level in your body. The variety of the delicious rainbow of foods you are eating should be making you feel alive, and you should have more energy. As we move through these next two weeks, you may get an energy boost as we reintroduce carbs, but, beware, hearty grains may initially shock your system.

Great job, you made it to the third week! This week you will experience a wide range of colors, flavors, and textures for a healthier, happier you. Continue to eat the foods allowed during week two. Use the alkaline/acid food chart to help you make the right choices when balancing your plate. Stay focused on finding foods that taste as great as they make you feel. Pick two new foods to try this week. This will help you conquer any cravings you are having.

The movement of the week is thirty minutes of exercise for five days; keep stretching for ten minutes before and after you exercise. Keep dancing. Make an appointment for a massage, or get into a sauna this week.

The affirmation of the week concerns your career or occupation. Remind yourself that a part of all you earn is yours to keep. This concept is based on the principle of paying yourself first to accumulate wealth. Save at least 10 percent of what you earn each week, and put it into a separate account. When you are ready to celebrate you, this money will be there for you to do whatever you want. This is a new, healthy mind-set habit. This is the third affirmation you can use every day.---"A part of all I earn is mine to keep" Keep writing the affirmations in your journal.

Your mindful meditation of the week is a visualization exercise. What does the end result of this program look like for you? How will the people in your life celebrate you? Is it just the desire to feel better in clothes? Be really clear about your goal; visualize every detail. Dig deeper and think about how it will really feel for you to succeed with this program. What will six months from now look like? What will one year look like?

Your journal writing for this week will be writing down your visualization exercise. Be clear. Each weekend journal about your greatest accomplishment for the week, the biggest challenge you had, and what your main health concerns are.

Week four is a big week; you are one more week away from completing the mindful-eating program. Revisit the health questionnaire you filled out at the beginning of the program. Over the past three weeks, you'll probably find you have lost some of those symptoms you listed and also that you have lost some weight, gained better sleep and increased energy, and have started thinking more clearly. Finish this last week strong, with no processed foods or drinks. If you eat animal proteins, it's OK to add those back on your plate, but do opt for organic/sustainable options when possible.

Let's talk about reintroducing foods to your clean, healthy, energized body. Don't go crazy and add in too many of the foods that you have been avoiding for the past three weeks. Go slowly, and reintroduce foods one by one; you will be able to see how your body responds. This process can be a helpful way to find out if you are sensitive to foods that cause inflammation and fatigue. If you find a food that definitely seems to cause symptoms, exclude it from your plate for two to three months, and then eat it again to see if you still have symptoms. Symptoms can be bloating, nausea, constipation, increased heart rate, unpleasant mood changes, depression, poor concentration, head-aches, fluid retention, lethargy, or joint aches or pains. If you experience no reaction, then move on with lunch and dinner. If you have a reaction, then immediately stop eating that food. Record all of your symptoms and your body's reactions to these foods. If you have a reaction, drink lots of water to flush out your system.

The movement of the week is thirty minutes of exercise for five days with ten minutes of stretching before and after exercise. Turn on the music, get up and dance! Have another massage and a sauna this week. Yoga is an amazing way to exercise; it's great for stress and weight loss. Yoga is a gentle exercise that can aid in eliminating waste, but to experience the benefits of yoga fully, you will need to attend a class.

The affirmation of the week is about your spiritual beliefs or practices. Say, "Thank you, _____ for blessing me with abundance every day in every way." This affirmation is very powerful, and you can actually give this one some rhythm.

During your journal writing this week, take a moment and check in with yourself. What are your intentions or goals for the upcoming days, weeks, and months of the year? What is good in your life right now, and what would you like to see change? Create two to five action steps to accomplish these goals or intentions. You will feel more centered and less stressed, and you will have more energy to create balance and enjoy your new, healthy lifestyle.

Phase Three—An Optional Phase

Phase three is the fasting phase. This phase can be the most challenging, but it can also be the most productive. Now that you have completed phases one and two, you should be ready for a one-to-three-day fast. I have included a seven-day fast, which can be modified for one to three days. Following the fasting, you will return to phase two, weeks three and four, of the program.

CHAPTER SIX

THE MINDFUL-EATING MEAL PROGRAM

"When you break a small habit, you teach yourself that you can change anything."—Unknown

During the coming weeks, you will learn ways to achieve a healthier lifestyle. You've got this! You have everything you need to push forward one day at a time. Spend each day noticing how certain foods feel in your body. Also pay attention to your emotional reactions and triggers.

Everyone is going to use the program a little bit differently because each of you is starting from a different place in life. You have your own set of health goals, and those may be different than someone else's. You only look at *you* in the mirror. You are your own best friend.

This Mindful-Eating Meal Program is pretty easy. You choose from the options of the weekly menu. Choose what you would like to eat each day before the program starts. Take your shopping list, and purchase what you will need for the week, and prepare your meals a few days before the program. Stick with the program, and you will see results.

Here are some tips to help you organize your day-to-day activities for a successful mindful-eating program.

1. Set goals. Use the handbook attached in this book, or go buy a journal. Write down three to five goals and what it would mean to you to have complete them.
2. Prepare the people in your life. Explain your eating plan to people you normally eat meals with; they should know how important this program is to you so they can support you.
3. Invite a friend to join you. Even the most motivated person can derail. If you do this program with a partner, you can encourage each other.
4. Drink plenty of water. The water you drink flushes out the toxins in your system, keeps hunger at bay, and keeps you hydrated. Start every morning with warm water and a squeeze of lemon.
5. Space out your meals by eating every four to five hours rather than nonstop nibbling. Evenly spaced meals will keep your metabolism even.
6. Keep track of what, when, and where you eat and the amount of liquids you are consuming, as well as how you feel before, during, and after you eat. This will bring awareness and transform your relationship with food.
7. Stick to each week's menu. Different phases of the program offer different foods for a reason, so don't jump ahead.
8. Use Saturday and Sunday to do your shopping and to prep food for the week. Clean any fresh fruit and vegetables. Prepare dishes for the coming week. This may sound like a lot of time spent cooking, but it will save you time during the week.
9. Please note that most dinners are designed so you can use leftovers for lunch the next day.

10. If you are feeling full or in a rush, know that you can exchange a meal for a smoothie as long as you put in a scoop of protein powder and crushed flaxseeds or chia seeds.
11. Eat slowly, and chew your food well—about thirty times.
12. Hydrate. Drink one-half your body weight in ounces of water each day. (For example, if your weight is two hundred pounds, drink one hundred ounces of water.)
13. Try to go to bed at least thirty minutes earlier than you normally would.

Tips for Eating Out

1. Always choose wild fish over farm-raised fish.
2. Always choose grass-fed beef.
3. You can ask to switch all side dishes to two vegetables, instead.
4. Always ask how the food is prepared.
5. Bring wheat-free pasta, and ask the chef to prepare it for you.
6. If you are not hungry, just order a few appetizers, or consider sharing an entrée.
7. Bring your own tea bag, and order a cup of hot water, or, instead of tea, order a cup of hot water with lemon.

Self-Care

Self-care is taking time out for you. Go ahead! Check your schedule. Make an appointment for yourself.

1. Have a gentle massage, reflexology, shiatsu, or any other type of bodywork to help increase circulation and aid in healing your body.
2. Dry brush your skin to help cleanse and stimulate your largest organ of elimination. Use a natural-bristle skin brush while your skin is dry, and begin with your feet, then move up toward your heart.

3. Deep-breathing exercises help to eliminate toxins through the lungs while calming and centering the mind and body.

4. Get outside for fifteen minutes, and allow your skin to absorb the sun.

5. Enjoy the amazing feeling of being alive, and be grateful for your life.

WEEK ONE—BREAKFAST

"Let food be thy medicine and medicine be thy food."—Hippocrates

*B*reakfast options are juices and smoothies. Add a tablespoon of ground flaxseed and a scoop of protein powder (no dairy, no soy) to each *smoothie.*

Carrot and Grapefruit Juice

> 2 grapefruits, peeled and with the pith removed
> 5 chopped carrots
> 1 inch of fresh ginger, peeled and chopped
> Press all ingredients into the juicer. Stir and serve immediately.

Apple and Beet Juice

> 1 chopped small beet
> 5 chopped carrots
> 1 cored and chopped apple
> ¼ cup of fresh mint sprigs.
> Press all ingredients into the juicer. Stir and serve immediately.

Green Lemonade

> ½ chopped lemon
> 2 cups baby spinach

1 chopped cucumber
2 cored and chopped sweet apples
Press all ingredients into the juicer. Stir and serve immediately.

Cucumber and Pear Juice

1 cored and chopped pear
1 inch sliced, fresh ginger
1 chopped cucumber
3 chopped stalks of celery
Press all the ingredients into the juicer. Stir and serve immediately.

Pineapple-Spinach Juice

1 cup baby spinach
5 cups chopped romaine lettuce leaves
3 cups chopped pineapple
Press all the ingredients into the juicer. Stir and serve immediately.

Green Island Smoothie

6 chopped romaine lettuce leaves
4 chopped kale leaves
½ cup fresh parsley sprigs
½ cup chopped, fresh pineapple
½ cup chopped, fresh mango
1 inch of fresh ginger, peeled and chopped
1 ½ cups water
Put all ingredients in a blender, and blend until smooth.

Blueberry-Mint Smoothie

1 cup frozen blueberries
½ avocado

¼ cup orange juice
½ cup fresh mint leaves
1 teaspoon lemon juice
½ cup water
Blend until smooth.

Sassy Mango Smoothie

1 cup frozen mango, slightly thawed
1 tablespoon tahini,
1 tablespoon lime juice
½ cup water
Blend until smooth.

$\mathcal{W}$EEK $\mathcal{O}$NE—$\mathcal{L}$UNCH

"Let food be thy medicine and medicine be thy food."—Hippocrates

Lunch options can be made ahead of time and refrigerated.

Roasted Beets on Greens—Makes four servings
Heat oven to 400 degrees.
Wrap two bunches of trimmed beets in foil, and roast until tender, about one hour.
Let cool, and then peel and dice. 2 cups baby spinach
½ cup chopped parsley leaves
1 red onion, sliced thinly
Whisk together…
3 tablespoons of extra-virgin olive oil (EVOO)
Juice of one lemon
2 teaspoons honey
1 minced clove garlic
1 teaspoon fennel seeds

Season with salt and pepper. Toss with beets. Toss one cup of the dressed beets with one cup baby spinach and one-fourth cup fresh parsley leaves, per serving. Top with thinly sliced red onion.

Kale Slaw with Red Cabbage and Carrot—Makes four servings
1 tablespoon EVOO

1 tablespoon Dijon Mustard
1 teaspoon apple-cider vinegar
1 ½ cups shredded kale
1 ½ cups shredded red cabbage
1 carrot, peeled and julienned
½ cup fresh parsely, chopped
2 tablespoons each, sunflower, pumpkin and hemp seeds

In a small bowl, whisk one tablespoon olive oil, one tablespoon Dijon mustard, and one teaspoon apple-cider vinegar. Season as desired.

In another bowl, combine three cups mixed shredded kale and red cabbage, one peeled and julienned carrot, one-fourth cup fresh parsley leaves, two tablespoons each of sunflower, pumpkin, and hemp seeds. Season as desired, then drizzle with dressing.

Spiced Butternut Squash Soup—Makes six servings
2 tablespoons EVOO
1 onion, chopped and diced
2 garlic cloves, chopped
Fresh ginger, 1 inch, grated
½ teaspoon turmeric
2 carrots, peeled and chopped
1 tart apple, cored, peeled and chopped
Butternut Squash, chopped
3 cups, water

Heat two tablespoons of olive oil over medium heat. Add one chopped onion and two chopped garlic cloves. Cook until tender, about six minutes. Add one inch of grated, fresh ginger (two tablespoons), one-half teaspoon turmeric, three dashes of cinnamon and cardamom, and a dash of ground cloves. Cook about one minute, and add two peeled and chopped carrots, one cored and peeled, chopped tart apple, four cups chopped butternut squash, and three cups of water. Bring to a boil; partially cover, and reduce to simmer. Season as desired. Cook until vegetables are tender, about twenty minutes. Let cool slightly. Working in batches, puree until smooth in blender.

<u>Cleansing Broth</u>
1 Onion, large
6 Carrots, chopped
½ head celery, chopped
½ head Garlic
2 Sweet potatoes, chopped
12 cups water
4 cups spinach
1 bunch fresh parsley

Chop one large onion, six chopped carrots, one-half head of chopped celery, one halved head garlic, and two chopped large sweet potatoes. Put them in a large pot with twelve cups of water, and bring to a boil. Reduce heat, and simmer for twenty minutes. Add four cups spinach and one bunch fresh parsley, and simmer five minutes. Season as desired. Strain liquid, and either discard vegetables or use the vegetables for a soup or stew. Broth will stay fresh up to five days in an airtight container.

<u>Super Easy Salad—Makes two servings</u>
4 cups mixed greens
½ cup carrots, shredded
½ cup red cabbage, shredded
½ cup zucchini, shredded
½ cup sprouts
¼ cup balsamic vinegar
4 to 8 oz of protein

Mix four cups of your favorite mixed greens, arugula, watercress, and/ or spinach with one-half cup shredded carrots, one-half cup shredded red cabbage, one-half cup shredded zucchini, and one-half cup of your favorite sprouts, or use any vegetables in your refrigerator. Use one-fourth cup balsamic vinaigrette for dressing. Add four to eight ounces of protein such as salmon or quinoa.

<u>Striped Bass with Fenne—Makes two servings</u>
1medium white onion
1 fennel bulb, sliced thin
½ lemon, juiced
(2) 4 to 8 oz filet striped bass
1 tablespoon capers
¼ cup Italian parsley, chopped

Slice one quarter of a medium white onion, and thinly slice a fennel bulb. Place the ingredients in a medium-sized saucepan and add the juice from half a lemon and about one inch of water. Bring to a boil, and simmer for five minutes. Remove from heat. Season the fish with sea salt, and put into the saucepan. Sprinkle one tablespoon of rinsed capers and one-fourth cup Italian parsley over the fish. Cover the saucepan with the lid. Simmer for about ten minutes, until the fish is almost flakey. To serve, place vegetables on the bottom of a shallow dish, and place the fish on top; drizzle with olive oil and fresh parsley.

WEEK ONE—DINNER

"Let food be thy medicine and medicine be thy food."—Hippocrates

Options can be made ahead of time and refrigerated.

Roasted Portobello Mushrooms with Kale—Makes two servings
¼ cup apple-cider vinegar
1 tablespoon honey
4 cloves garlic
2 tablespoon EVOO
4 portobello mushrooms
1 red onion, thinly sliced
red pepper flakes, pinch
6 cups kale, thinly sliced

Heat oven to 400 degrees. Combine one-fourth cup of apple-cider vinegar, one tablespoon honey, two chopped cloves of garlic, and one tablespoon EVOO in a bowl. Season as desired. Arrange four stemmed portobello mushrooms in a baking dish. Drizzle the vinaigrette over the mushrooms. Cover and marinate for at least thirty minutes or overnight in the refrigerator. In a large skillet, heat one tablespoon of oil over medium heat. Add one-half of a thinly sliced red onion, two thinly sliced cloves of garlic, and a pinch of red pepper flakes. Cook until softened, about five minutes. Add six cups thinly sliced kale. Season with salt, and cook covered about four minutes. Roast mushrooms, flipping once after about thirty minutes. Serve topped with kale.

Red-Lentil and Sweet-Potato Stew—Makes four servings
2 tablespoons of coconut oil or EVOO
1 teaspoon each of ground cumin and turmeric
1 tablespoon of curry powder
1 onion, diced
4 cloves of garlic
2 tablespoons fresh ginger, minced
2 sweet potatoes, peeled and diced
1 red bell pepper, cleaned and diced
1 ½ cups red lentils, rinsed
6 cups cleansing broth
¼ bunch fresh cilantro

Heat two tablespoons of coconut oil or EVOO in a large pot, over medium heat. Add one teaspoon each of ground cumin and turmeric and one tablespoon of curry powder. Heat for about one to two minutes. Add one large, diced onion with a few pinches of salt. Cook until tender, about six minutes. Add four minced cloves of garlic and two tablespoons minced fresh ginger, and cook until tender, about two minutes. Add two peeled and diced sweet potatoes and one cleaned and diced red bell pepper. Cook for a minute. Add one and one-half cups rinsed red lentils and six cups of cleansing broth (see recipe). Bring to boil, then reduce heat, and simmer until lentils are tender, about twenty to twenty-five minutes. Season as desired. Top with fresh, chopped cilantro.

Steamed Broccoli and Squash with Tahini Sauce—Makes four servings
½ head of broccoli
1 delicata squash
1 cup mixed greens
1 cup red cabbage, thinly sliced

½ red onion, diced
Tahini sauce
1 tablespoon sesame seeds, toasted

Steam one-half head of broccoli florets about four minutes. Remove from pan, and set aside. Steam one sliced and seeded delicata squash about ten minutes. In a bowl, toss one cup mixed greens, one cup thinly sliced red cabbage and two tablespoons diced red onion. Top with steamed vegetables. Season as desired. Drizzle with tahini sauce (see recipe below), and sprinkle with one tablespoon toasted sesame seeds.

Tahini Sauce
½ cup tahini
1 lemon, juiced
1 tablespoon EVOO
1 garlic clove
½ teaspoon cumin
½ teaspoon paprika
¾ cup water

In a food processor, puree one-half cup tahini, the grated zest and juice of one lemon, one tablespoon olive oil, one chopped garlic clove, one-half teaspoon cumin, one-half teaspoon paprika, and three-fourths of a cup water until smooth. Season with salt.

Carrot Ginger Soup—Makes four servings
2 tablespoons EVOO
1 shallot, minced
2 tablespoons fresh ginger, minced
1 pound carrots, peeled and chopped
2 cups vegetable or chicken broth
½ teaspoon salt
¼ teaspoon coriander
2 green onions

Pour a small amount of EVOO in a pan, and heat on a medium-high setting. Add minced shallot, and sauté until tender. Add two tablespoons minced fresh ginger, and sauté. Add one pound carrots, peeled and chopped, two cups vegetable or chicken broth, one-half teaspoon salt, and one-fourth teaspoon coriander. Reduce heat to simmer, and cook ten to fifteen minutes, until carrots are tender. Carefully transfer to blender and puree. Top with thinly sliced green onions, and serve.

If you don't feel great, and you do not have lots of energy after week one, you may need to repeat week one. That's all right; everyone is different. If this is the case for you, just repeat week one and then move on to week two.

WEEK
TWO—BREAKFAST

Focus on awareness of your food.

Try these recipes, or you can also use any of the week one recipes.

<u>Cardamom Quinoa Porridge—Makes two servings</u>
½ cup quinoa, rinsed
¾ cup unsweetened almond milk
½ cup water
½ teaspoon vanilla extract
¼ teaspoon coarse salt
¼ teaspoon cardamom
½ pear
2 tablespoons almonds, sliced

In a saucepan, bring to boil one-half cup rinsed quinoa, three-fourths cup unsweetened almond milk, one-half cup water, one-half teaspoon vanilla extract, one-fourth teaspoon coarse salt, and one-fourth teaspoon ground cardamom. Reduce heat, cover, and simmer until liquid is absorbed, about fifteen minutes. Remove from heat; fluff, and let sit five minutes. Top each serving with a splash of almond milk, half a pear (sliced), and two tablespoons sliced almonds.

Banana-Oat Pancakes—Makes two servings
1 banana
½ cup unsweetened almond milk
3 tablespoons flaxseed meal
3 tablespoons coconut oil
½ cup oat flour
½ cup unsweetened shredded coconut
¼ cup orange juice
½ teaspoon baking powder
½ teaspoon cinnamon
Coarse salt
Fresh orange
Local honey

In a bowl, combine half a banana (mashed), one-half cup unsweetened almond milk, three tablespoons flaxseed meal, and two teaspoons coconut oil. Let stand until thick, about ten minutes. Whisk in one-half cup oat flour, one-half cup unsweetened shredded coconut, one-fourth cup orange juice, one-half teaspoon baking powder, one-half teaspoon ground cinnamon, and a pinch of coarse salt. Heat two tablespoons of coconut oil in a cast-iron skillet over medium heat. Working in batches, spoon in one-fourth cup of batter, and cook each pancake about six minutes per side. (You may have to gently flatten the pancakes while they are cooking.) Serve with orange segments and honey.

Vegetable Soup with Chickpeas and Miso—Makes four servings
2 tablespoons EVOO
1 yellow onion
2 garlic cloves
2 celery stalks, diced
2 carrots, peeled and diced
1 cup broccoli, chopped
1 cup chickpeas
2 tablespoons white miso

Heat two tablespoons of olive oil in a pot, over medium heat. Cook one-half chopped yellow onion, two minced garlic cloves, two diced celery stalks, and two peeled and diced carrots for six to eight minutes. Stir in one cup chopped broccoli and one cup chickpeas. Cook two minutes. Add four cups of water. Bring to a boil. Reduce heat, and simmer for ten minutes. Remove from heat. Dissolve two tablespoons white miso into two tablespoons cool water, and stir into soup.

Baked Sweet Potatoes with Toasted Nuts and Oranges—Makes two servings

2 sweet potatoes
¼ cup almonds or pecans, chopped and toasted
Dash of cinnamon, freshly grated nutmeg and sea salt.
1 fresh orange

Heat oven to 400 degrees. Prick two small sweet potatoes with a fork, and wrap them in foil. Bake until tender, about one hour. Unwrap, and split with a knife. Top with one-fourth cup chopped, toasted almonds or pecans, a dash of cinnamon, a dash of freshly grated nutmeg, and sea salt. Serve with two orange wedges.

$\mathcal{W}$EEK $\mathcal{T}$WO—$\mathcal{L}$UNCH

Focus on awareness of your food.

(You can also use any of the recipes from week one.)

<u>Broccoli and Chickpea Salad</u>—Makes four servings
4 cups broccoli florets
1 15oz can chickpeas, drained and rinsed
5 scallions
½ cup fresh parsley, chopped
1/3 cup pine nuts, toasted
1 clove garlic, minced
2 teaspoons Dijon mustard
1 teaspoon local honey
1 tablespoon lemon zest, grated
¼ cup lemon juice
6 tablespoons EVOO

Steam four cups of broccoli florets until tender, five to seven minutes. Cool the broccoli, then chop it, and combine with a fifteen ounce can of drained and rinsed chickpeas. Also add five sliced scallions, one-half cup chopped fresh parsley, and one-third cup toasted pine nuts. In a bowl, combine one minced clove of garlic, two teaspoons Dijon mustard, one teaspoon honey, one tablespoon grated lemon zest, and one-fourth cup lemon juice. Slowly add six tablespoons EVOO, whisking to emulsify, and season with coarse sea salt and freshly ground black pepper. Drizzle the broccoli mixture with dressing.

Lemon-Herb Sardine Salad—Makes two servings
2 tablespoons EVOO
1 teaspoon lemon zest
1 lemon, juiced
1 teaspoon Dijon mustard
1 tablespoon capers, rinsed
2 tablespoons fresh parsley
1 tablespoon fresh tarragon
2 celery stalks
(2) 4.4 ounce olive-oil packed sardines
Mixed greens

Combine the following ingredients in a bowl: two tablespoons EEVO, one teaspoon grated lemon zest, the juice of one lemon, one teaspoon Dijon mustard, one tablespoon rinsed capers, two tablespoons chopped, fresh parsley, one tablespoon chopped, fresh tarragon, and two finely diced stalks of celery. Gently fold in two 4.4–ounce cans of olive-oil-packed sardines, and season as desired. Serve on lettuce.

Baked Sweet Potatoes with Greens—Makes two servings
2 sweet potatoes
1 tablespoon EVOO
1 onion, sliced thinly
1 bunch Swiss chard, stemmed and chopped
1 avocado
Dashes of cayenne, salt
1 lemon, squeezed

Heat oven to 400 degrees. Prick two sweet potatoes; wrap them in foil, and bake about forty-five minutes. Heat one tablespoon EVOO in a large skillet over medium heat. Add one thinly sliced small onion, and cook about six minutes. Add one stemmed and chopped bunch of Swiss chard, and cook, stirring until the Swiss chard is bright green and wilted, about five minutes. Split the potatoes, and top each with the greens and one-half sliced avocado. Season with cayenne, salt, and a squeeze of lemon.

Raw Kale Salad with Pomegranate and Toasted Walnuts—Makes four servings
1 bunch kale
2 tablespoons EVOO
1 tablespoon fresh lime juice
½ teaspoon fresh ginger, grated
½ cup pomegrante seeds
1 red onion
¼ cup walnuts, chopped and toasted

Rub one bunch of torn kale with two tablespoons EVOO, one tablespoon fresh lime juice, and one-half teaspoon freshly grated ginger until well coated. Add one-half cup pomegranate seeds (from half a pomegranate), two tablespoons chopped red onion, and one-fourth cup chopped, toasted walnuts. Toss all the ingredients together, and season to taste.

Watercress with Sardines, Tarragon, and Orange Citrus—Makes two servings
1 lemon
1 tablespoon EVOO
2 cups watercress
1 red onion
1 tablespoon fresh tarragon
1 fresh orange
1 4 ounce can olive-oil packed sardines
3 tablespoons pumpkin seeds, toasted

Whisk zest and the juice of half a lemon with one tablespoon EVOO. Season with coarse salt and pepper. Arrange two cups of watercress sprigs, one-fourth of a small red onion, sliced, and one tablespoon of freshly chopped tarragon on a plate. Top with slices of peeled orange citrus. Drain one four-ounce can of olive-oil-packed sardines. Place the sardines and three tablespoons of toasted pumpkin seeds on top of the orange citrus. Season with coarse salt and pepper, and drizzle with vinaigrette.

<u>Red Lentil Soup with Turnip and Parsley</u>—Makes eight servings
2 tablespoons EVOO
1 yellow onion
4 garlic cloves
3 celery stalks, diced finely
1 ½ cups tomatoes, chopped
1 ½ cups dried red lentils
1 turnip, peeled and diced
6 cups water
½ cup fresh parsley, chopped
1 teaspoon red-wine vinegar

Heat two tablespoons of EVOO in a pot, over medium heat. Add one diced yellow onion, four minced garlic cloves, and three finely diced celery stalks. Cook until tender, six to eight minutes. Increase heat to high, and add one and one-half cups chopped tomatoes; cook for a minute. Add one and one-half cups dried red lentils, one peeled and diced turnip, and six cups water. Bring to a boil, then reduce heat, and simmer for twenty to twenty-five minutes. Stir in one-half cup chopped, fresh flat-leaf parsley and, if you like, one teaspoon of red-wine vinegar. Season with salt and pepper.

Here are some tips for week two. If you are feeling hungry, it might be your body telling you it's dehydrated. Drink a glass of water, and wait twenty minutes before eating your next meal.

$\mathcal{W}$EEK $\mathcal{T}$WO—$\mathcal{D}$INNER

Focus on awareness of your food.

In addition to these recipes, you can also use the recipes from week one.

<u>Roasted Winter Vegetables with Cannellini Beans-Makes four servings</u>
1 large leek
5 garlic cloves
1 rutabaga, peeled and chopped
2 parsnips, peeled and chopped
2 carrots, peeled and chopped
1 sweet potato, peeled and chopped
8 brussels sprouts
3 tablespoons EVOO
2 tablespoon balsamic vinegar
1 ½ cups cannellini beans, cooked and drained

Heat the oven to 425 degrees. Grab a baking sheet, and put the following ingredients on it: one sliced, large leek, five peeled garlic cloves, one-half peeled and chopped small rutabaga, two peeled, chopped parsnips, two peeled and chopped carrots, one peeled and chopped sweet potato, and eight trimmed and halved brussels sprouts with three tablespoons of EVOO and one tablespoon of balsamic vinegar. Season as desired. Roast the vegetables until tender (tossing once), about twenty-five to thirty minutes.

Remove from oven, and stir in one and one-half cups cooked and drained cannellini beans. Cook until the beans are crisped, about fifteen minutes more. Toss vegetables with one teaspoon vinegar, and drizzle with oil.

Grilled Salmon and Bok Choy with Avocado Salsa-Makes two servings
1 navel orange
1 avocado
1 tablespoon red onion, chopped
1 tablespoon fresh cilantro, chopped
1 teaspoon lime juice
¼ teaspoon toasted sesame oil
(2) 4 ounch filet wild salmon
3 heads bok choy

Heat a grill or grill pan to medium high.
In a medium bowl, combine segments from one navel orange, one-half diced avocado, one tablespoon Chopped red onion, one tablespoon freshly chopped cilantro, one teaspoon lime juice, and one-fourth teaspoon toasted sesame oil. Season as desired, and set aside. Season two four-ounce fillets of wild salmon and three heads of bok choy (halved) with salt and pepper, and drizzle with EVOO. Grill salmon, cooking three to four minutes per side. Grill bok choy until bright green, about two minutes per side. Spoon avocado salsa over fish to serve.

Roasted Vegetables with Quinoa-Makes two servings
2 cups butternut squash, diced
1 cup carrots, diced
1 sweet potato, peeled and diced
1 cup brussel sprouts, trimmed and halved
2 tablespoons coconut oil or EVOO
1 teaspoon smoked paprika
1 cup quinoa, cooked

1 ½ cups baby spinach
Sauce:
1 garlic clove
2 tablespoons tahini
3 tablespoons apple-cider vinegar
2 tablespoons EVOO
¼ cup each fresh chives, parsley and cilantro

Heat oven to 425 degrees.
Toss two cups of diced butternut squash, one cup of carrots, one sweet potato (peeled and diced), and one cup trimmed and halved brussels sprouts with two tablespoons melted coconut oil or EVOO. Season with salt and one teaspoon smoked paprika. Roast, rotating the pan occasionally, until the vegetables are tender, about twenty-five to thirty minutes. Make the sauce by pulsing the following ingredients in a food processor, until smooth: one garlic clove, two tablespoons tahini, three tablespoons apple-cider vinegar, two tablespoons EVOO, two tablespoons water, and one-fourth cup each chopped fresh chives, parsley, and cilantro. Season as desired. In a large bowl, toss roasted vegetables with one cup cooked quinoa and two tablespoons sauce. Toss each serving with one and one-fourth cups baby spinach.

<u>Baked Salmon with Coconut Broth-Makes two servings</u>
1 clove garlic
1 small red chili
1 stalk lemongrass
1 cup coconut milk
(2) 5 ounce skinless, wild salmon fillets
2 tablespoon EVOO
½ red onion, sliced
1 cup carrots, thinly sliced
1 head baby bok-choy, sliced
½ cup cooked brown rice

2 scallions
1 lime

In a small pot, combine and bring to a boil the following ingredients:
1 smashed clove garlic, ½ thinly sliced small red chili
1 chopped stalk lemongrass (outer layers removed)
½ cup cleansing broth (see recipe)
1 cup coconut milk

Reduce heat and simmer until fragrant, about twenty minutes. Strain and discard solids. Keep warm. Heat oven to 375 degrees.

Rub two five-ounce, skinless wild salmon fillets with one tablespoon EVOO, and season with coarse salt. Bake until just cooked through, ten minutes. Meanwhile, heat one tablespoon EVOO in a skillet over medium heat. Add one-half sliced red onion, one cup thinly sliced carrots, and one sliced head of baby bok choy. Cook, stirring until tender, about five minutes.

For each serving, top one-half cup cooked brown rice with salmon fillet and vegetables.

Ladle broth over the dinner, and garnish with sliced scallions and a squeeze of lime.

Baked Trout with Broccoli, Apple, and Fennel Slaw-Makes four servings

4 trout fillets
Coarse salt and freshly ground pepper
Extra-virgin olive oil, for drizzling
1 lemon, thinly sliced
1 shallot, thinly sliced
1 tablespoon tahini
1 teaspoon grated lemon zest, plus 1 tablespoon lemon juice
1 tablespoon apple sauce
3 broccoli stalks, peeled and julienned (about 1 1/2 cup)
1/2 bulb fennel, thinly sliced
1 carrot, peeled and julienned

1/2 tart apple, peeled, cored, and julienned
2 tablespoons chopped fresh parsley

Preheat oven to 400 degrees. Cut four pieces of parchment paper to twelve by sixteen inches, and arrange one fish fillet in the center of each piece. Season with salt and pepper, and top with lemon slices and shallot. Drizzle with olive oil. To fold parchment join the long sides together, and make a few quarter-inch folds to seal. Fold the ends like you're wrapping a gift, and tuck them underneath. Transfer parchments packets to a rimmed baking sheet. Bake until packet is puffed and fish is cooked through, twelve to fourteen minutes. Remove from oven, and let rest five minutes. In a medium bowl, whisk together tahini, lemon zest and juice, applesauce, and one tablespoon water. Season with salt. Stir in broccoli, fennel, carrot, apple, and parsley until combined. Serve slaw with fish.

WEEK THREE — BREAKFAST

Make it last; form healthy habits.

<u>Roasted Red Pepper and Kale Frittata-Makes one serving</u>
1 tablespoon EVOO
1 scallion, sliced
1 cup chopped kale
¼ cup roasted red pepper, diced
2 organic large eggs

Heat oven to 350 degrees.
In a small, ovenproof skillet, heat one tablespoon EVOO on medium heat on the stove.
Add one sliced scallion and one cup chopped kale, and cook, stirring until just wilted, about two minutes. Add one-fourth cup diced, roasted red pepper, and cook until heated through. Season with coarse salt and freshly cracked ground pepper. Pour two whisked large eggs over vegetables, and transfer skillet to oven. Bake until eggs are cooked through, about five minutes.

<u>Banana-Apple Buckwheat Muffins-Makes four muffins</u>
¼ cup buckwheat flour
1 teaspoon baking powder

½ teaspoon ground cinnamon
1/8 teaspoon coarse salt
2 organic eggs
1 banana
¼ cup local honey
1 sweet apple, cored, peeled, finely diced
¼ cup walnuts

Heat oven to 350 degrees.
Place four baking cups in a muffin tin.
In a bowl whisk together one-fourth cup buckwheat flour, one teaspoon baking powder, one-half teaspoon ground cinnamon, and one-eighth teaspoon coarse salt. In another bowl whisk together two large eggs, one-half of a mashed banana, and one-fourth cup honey. Mix the wet ingredients into the dry ones, and then fold in half of a sweet apple (peeled, cored, and finely diced) and one-fourth cup chopped walnuts. Fill the baking cups with batter, and fill the empty cups of the baking tin halfway with water. Bake thirty minutes or until a tester comes out clean. Let cool on a wire rack.

Toasted Coconut Muesli-Makes one serving
2 tablespoons unsweetened coconut flakes, toasted
2 tablespoons gluten-free rolled oats
1 apple
¼ cup fresh berries
¼ cup almond milk
In a bowl combine two tablespoons of toasted, unsweetened coconut flakes, two tablespoons of gluten-free rolled oats, half an apple (sliced), one-fourth cup fresh berries, and one-fourth cup almond milk.

Steamed Salmon with Herbs and Lemon-Makes one serving
(1) 4 ounce wild-salmon fillet
½ cup cooked brown rice

Fresh herbs, dill parsley, chives
1 lemon to zest

Season one four-ounce wild-salmon fillet with coarse salt and pepper. Steam until just cooked through, eight minutes. Serve with one-half cup cooked brown rice. Sprinkle with fresh, chopped herbs (dill, parsley, chives) and lemon zest.

WEEK THREE—LUNCH

Make it last; form healthy habits.

Chickpea/Brown-Rice Veggie Burgers-Makes four servings
(1) 15 ounce can chickpeas, rinsed, cooked and drained
1 cup cooked brown rice
1 shallot, minced
1 clove garlic, minced
2 tablespoons fresh parsley
1 organic egg
2 tablespoons EVOO
Whole-grain mustard
1 red onion
1 roasted red-pepper
leaf lettuce

Mash two cups of cooked and drained chickpeas and one cup of cooked brown rice until a thick paste forms. Stir in one minced shallot, one minced garlic clove, and two tablespoons chopped, fresh parsley. Season to taste. Stir in one whisked, large egg. Form into four one-half-inch-thick patties. Heat two tablespoons of EVOO in a large skillet over medium heat. Add patties, and cook until golden brown, about four minutes per side. Spread with whole-grain mustard, slices of red onion, and roasted red pepper, and wrap in a leaf of lettuce.

Rice Noodles with Broccoli-Almond Pesto-Makes four servings
1 head broccoli
7 tablespoons almonds, sliced and toasted
¼ cup fresh basil leaves
1 clove garlic
2 tablespoons lemon juice
6 tablespoons EVOO
Rice noodles

Bring a medium-sized pot of well-salted water to a boil. Cook one head of broccoli florets and sliced stems until tender, about two minutes. Remove the broccoli with a slotted spoon, and let cool slightly. (Reserve water.) Coarsely chop one cup cooked florets, and set aside. Puree remaining florets, six tablespoons of sliced, toasted almonds, one-fourth cup fresh basil leaves, one minced garlic clove, and two tablespoons lemon juice. Add six tablespoons of EVOO. Season to taste, and set aside.

Return water to boil, and cook eight ounces of medium rice noodles according to package instructions. Reserve one cup of the cooking water; drain noodles, and return them to the pot.

Toss with pesto, adding reserved pasta water until creamy. Top each bowl with chopped florets, small basil leaves, and remaining almonds. Season to taste.

Avocado and Black Bean Tacos-Makes one serving
1 avocado
1 clove garlic
1 tablespoon lime juice
Dash of cumin
Corn tortilla's
½ cup kale, thinly sliced
¼ cup black beans, cooked
2 tablespoons sunflower seeds, toasted

In a medium bowl, mash one-half avocado with one-half minced garlic clove, one tablespoon lime juice, and a dash of cumin. Season to taste. Toast two corn tortillas. Divide avocado mixture between tortillas, and top with one-half cup thinly sliced kale, one-fourth cup cooked black beans, and two tablespoons toasted sunflower seeds.

Stuffed Acorn Squash-Makes two servings
1 acorn squash
2 ½ tablespoons EVOO
1 large onion
1 teaspoon fresh sage, chopped
1 teaspoon fresh thyme
1/3 cup quinoa, cooked
1 cup kale, chopped
1 tablespoon hazelnuts, chopped and toasted
1 lemon

Heat oven to 400 degrees.
Brush one halved and seeded acorn squash with one teaspoon EVOO, and season with coarse salt and pepper. Roast cut-side down until tender, about thirty minutes. Flip and set aside.
Heat one tablespoons EVOO in a medium skillet over medium heat. Add one diced, large onion and cook, stirring until tender, about six minutes. Add one teaspoon chopped, fresh sage, one teaspoon fresh thyme, one-third cup cooked quinoa, and one cup chopped kale. Cook, stirring until greens wilt, about two minutes. Season with salt and pepper. Divide stuffing between squash halves, and roast until golden, fifteen to twenty minutes. Sprinkle each serving with one tablespoon chopped toasted hazelnuts. Drizzle with one tablespoon EVOO and squeezed lemon.

Quinoa Tabbouleh-Makes two servings
1 cup quinoa, rinsed
2 cups water or vegetable broth
½ teaspoon sea salt

1/3 cup fresh parsley,
3 green scallions

For this recipe you will need one cup quinoa, rinsed well, two cups water or vegetable broth, one-half teaspoon sea salt, one-third cup fresh parsley, minced, and three green scallions, minced.

In a saucepan combine the quinoa, water, and sea salt. Bring to a boil; reduce heat, and simmer until tender, about twenty minutes. Allow to cool. Once the quinoa has cooled a bit, add the parsley, green scallions, and lemon dressing. (See following recipe.) Toss well.

Lemon Dressing
¼ cup EVOO
Juice of one fresh lemon
Sea salt
1 clove garlic, pressed

Combine all the ingredients in a jar, and shake well. Pour over tabbouleh.

Halibut with Sweet-Potato Fries and Lime-Makes two servings
Work pure cooking techniques into your regular routine. Steaming, cooking *en papillote* (in parchment), and poaching all preserve flavor and nutrients.

2 sweet potatoes, peeled and cut into one-inch wedges
2 tablespoons extra-virgin olive oil
Coarse salt and freshly ground pepper
2 (4-ounce) halibut fillets, skin removed
1 tablespoon freshly chopped parsley
Lime wedges, for serving

Heat oven to 425 degrees. On a rimmed baking sheet, toss sweet potatoes with one tablespoon oil. Season with salt and pepper. Roast, tossing occasionally, until golden and tender, twenty minutes. During the last ten minutes of cooking, brush fish with remaining oil, and season with salt and pepper. Roast on a second baking sheet until cooked through, eight to ten minutes. Squeeze lime over fish and roasted sweet potatoes, and sprinkle with parsley.

Make it last; form healthy habits.

<u>Poached Egg with Rice and Edamame-Makes one Serving</u>
1 tablespoon EVOO
1 clove garlic
pinch red-pepper flakes
2 cups kale, chopped
½ cup frozen edamame beans
¾ cup brown rice, cooked
¼ cup red cabbage, shredded
1 organic egg

In a medium skillet, heat one tablespoon EVOO over medium heat. Add 1 clove sliced garlic and a pinch of red-pepper flakes. Cook about thirty seconds. Add two cups of chopped kale, and cook about two minutes. Add one-half cup thawed frozen edamame beans, and cook until heated through. Season to taste. Transfer to bowl with Put three-fourths of a cup of cooked brown rice in a bowl. Pour the kale and beans on top of the rice, and top that with one-fourth cup shredded red cabbage. In a small pot bring two inches of water to a boil, and then reduce it to a simmer.
Crack one large egg into a teacup, and gently slide the egg into the hot water. Cook until white is just set but yolk is still loose, three to four

minutes. Remove the egg with a slotted spoon and serve over rice and vegetables. Season to taste.

Spinach and Brown-Rice Bowl-Makes one serving
½ cup brown rice, cooked
2 teaspoons ginger, freshly grated
1 clove garlic, minced
3 cups water
½ cup baby spinach
1 scallion
1 tablespoon sesame seeds, toasted
4 to 8 ounces of protein, if desired-see approved foods list

In a small saucepan, bring to a boil one-half cup cooked, brown rice, two teaspoons freshly grated ginger, one clove minced garlic, and three cups of water. Cook, stirring occasionally, until thickened, about twenty-five minutes. Season to taste. Top with one-half cup baby spinach, one thinly sliced scallion, and one tablespoon toasted sesame seeds. Add four to eight ounces of protein, if desire.

Steamed Broccoli and Squash with Tahini Sauce-Makes four servings
1 head of broccoli
1 delicate squash
Mixed greens
1 cup red cabbage, sliced thinly
1 red onion
¼ cup tahini sauce
1 tablespoon sesame seeds, toasted

Steam one-half head of broccoli florets until they are bright green and tender, about four minutes. Remove and set aside. Steam one sliced and seeded delicate squash until it is bright yellow and tender, about ten minutes. Toss together the following ingredients in a bowl: one cup mixed greens, one cup thinly sliced red cabbage, and two tablespoons diced red onion. Top with steamed vegetables. Season to taste. Drizzle with one-fourth cup tahini sauce (recipe following), and sprinkle with one tablespoon toasted sesame seeds.

Tahini Sauce

In a food processor, puree until smooth, one-half cup tahini, grated zest and juice of one lemon, one tablespoon olive oil, one clove chopped garlic, one-half teaspoon cumin, one-half teaspoon paprika, and three-fourths of a cup water. Season to taste. Store sauce in airtight container up to one week.

Roasted Garlic Beet Soup-Makes four servings
3 red beets, medium size
6 garlic cloves
2 tablespoons EVOO
1 large leek
1 teaspoon fresh thyme
1 bay leaf
3 cups water
2 tablespoons freshly squeezed lemon juice

Heat oven to 400 degrees. Drizzle three medium beets with EVOO, and roast until tender, about an hour. Drizzle six unpeeled garlic cloves with EVOO, and roast in separate foil packet about thirty minutes. Unwrap beets. Let cool. Peel and quarter. Squeeze garlic from skin, and set aside.
Heat two tablespoons EVOO in a pot over medium heat. Add one thinly sliced large leek and cook, stirring until tender, seven minutes. Add beets and garlic, one teaspoon fresh thyme, one bay leaf, and three cups water. Bring to boil; reduce heat, and simmer for five minutes. Discard the bay leaf. Let the soup cool, and then puree in a blender until smooth. Stir in two tablespoons lemon juice, and season to taste.

Baked Cod with Lemon and EVOO-Makes four servings
(4) 4 to 6 ounces cod fillets
1 ½ tablespoons lemon juice, freshly squeezed
1 tablespoon olive oil
2 garlic cloves, minced
½ teaspoon thyme, dried
pinch of sea salt
¼ teaspoon paprika

Preheat oven to 400 degrees. Arrange four cod fillets (four to six ounces each) in a nine-by-thirteen-inch baking dish. Drizzle with one and one-half tablespoons freshly squeezed lemon juice and one tablespoon olive oil. Lightly rub in two cloves minced garlic, one-half teaspoon dried thyme, a pinch of sea salt, freshly ground black pepper, and one-fourth teaspoon of paprika. Bake for fifteen to twenty minutes until cod flesh is opaque but still juicy.

Steamed Bass with Fennel, Parsley, and Capers—Makes two servings
This recipe makes two servings, so you can share with a friend, keep one portion for the next day, or halve the recipe.

1/4 medium white onion, sliced
1 fennel bulb, thinly sliced
1/2 lemon, juice
2 5-ounce portions of striped bass
1/2 teaspoon sea salt
1 tablespoon capers, rinsed
1/4 cup Italian parsley, chopped
2 tablespoons extra-virgin olive oil

Additional olive oil and chopped fresh parsley, for garnish

Put onion, fennel, and lemon juice in a medium saucepan, and cover with one inch of water. Bring to a boil, and simmer for five minutes.

Remove from heat, and add in the two portions of fish, seasoned with sea salt. Sprinkle with capers and parsley, and cover the pan with a lid. Simmer for about nine minutes, until fish is almost flaky. Place the vegetables in the bottom of a shallow bowl and the fish on top; drizzle with olive oil, and sprinkle with fresh parsley. Serve one cup of steamed, brown rice per person on the side, if desired.

WEEK
FOUR—BREAKFAST

"If we eat wrongly, no doctors can cure us; if we eat rightly, no doctor is needed."—Victor G. Rocine

Black Quinoa Breakfast Cereal—Makes two servings
Black quinoa, like red quinoa, has a firmer texture than the white variety and makes a great alternative to breakfast cereal. Soft avocado provides a great contrast.

2 cups water
1/4 teaspoon salt
1 cup black quinoa
1 1/2 cups almond milk
1 thinly sliced avocado
6 tablespoons sliced toasted almonds
6 tablespoons honey

Bring two cups of water and salt to a boil. Whisk in quinoa. Return to a boil.
Reduce heat to low. Simmer, covered, for sixteen minutes. Let stand for five minutes.
Fluff with a fork, and top with almond milk, avocado, almonds, and honey.

Watercress with Garlic and Scrambled Eggs—Makes one serving
This zesty combo of fresh watercress, garlic, and scrambled eggs puts
a flavorful spin on any morning meal.

1 teaspoon olive oil
1 clove garlic, minced
1 cup watercress, stems removed
2 large organic eggs

Coarse salt and freshly ground black pepper
Heat one teaspoon of oil in a small skillet over medium heat. Add one
clove minced garlic, and cook until fragrant, about one minute. Add
watercress, and cook, stirring, until just wilted.
Remove from pan, and set aside. Turn heat down to medium low. Whisk
eggs, and season with salt and pepper. Pour eggs into pan, and cook, stirring, until just set. Return watercress to pan, and stir. Serve immediately.

Fresh Fruit with Applesauce-Sweetened Tahini—Makes one serving
Tahini and coconut give classic fruit salad an exotic twist. Mango,
grapes, and citrus fruit work well here, but you can also use any fruit
that's in season.

1/4 cup tahini
1/2 cup unsweetened applesauce
1 tablespoon honey
2 tablespoons water
4 cups sliced fruit, such as mango, black grapes, plums, and citrus
1/4 cup toasted, unsweetened coconut flakes

Combine tahini, applesauce, honey, and water in a food processor.
Pulse until smooth.
Arrange fruit in serving bowls. Drizzle with tahini sauce, and top with
toasted coconut.

Quinoa with Poached Egg, Spinach and Cucumber—Makes two servings

Quinoa (an ancient seed) is an excellent source of protein and contains all nine essential amino acids, making it a complete protein, like eggs. Eggs are the best natural source of the nutrient choline and help fight inflammation.

3 tablespoons olive oil
1 garlic clove, sliced
5 ounces spinach, rinsed
Coarse salt
1 carrot, peeled and julienned
2 large, organic eggs
1 1/2 cups cooked quinoa
1/4 cucumber, thinly sliced
1 teaspoon white-wine vinegar
Red-chili flakes
1 teaspoon minced chives

Heat one tablespoon of olive oil in a skillet over medium heat. Add garlic and cook, about one minute. Add spinach and steam, covered, until wilted, about one minute. Season with salt. Transfer to plate. Rinse pan, and fill with two inches of water; bring to a boil. Add carrot and cook until tender, about one minute. Transfer to plate. Reduce heat to a simmer, and poach eggs, three to four minutes. Divide quinoa between bowls. Top with egg, spinach, carrot, and cucumber. Whisk vinegar and two tablespoons of olive oil; season with salt. Drizzle over bowls of quinoa. Sprinkle with red-chili flakes and chives.

Avocado-Vanilla Smoothie

Now that you've made it this far, it's time to transform your relationship with food for life by keeping up the momentum this week. Start your day off with a creamy, guilt-free smoothie.

1 ripe avocado
1 cup no-sugar-added pear nectar, add more nectar as needed
1/2 teaspoon pure vanilla extract
1 cup ice cubes

Puree ingredients in a blender until smooth. If the smoothie is too thick, add more nectar to adjust consistency.

ᏔᎬᎬᏦ ᏚᎾᏌᏒ—ᎬᏌᏁᏟᎻ

"If we eat wrongly, no doctors can cure us; if we eat rightly, no doctor is needed."—Victor G. Rocine

Quinoa Salad with Toasted Almonds—Makes two servings
Quinoa, which is used like a grain but is really a seed, can be found at natural foods stores and many supermarkets.

1/4 cup slivered almonds
1/2 cup (3 ounces) quinoa
4 teaspoons olive oil
1 yellow bell pepper, ribs and seeds discarded, cut into 1/2-inch chunks
2 garlic cloves, minced
2 scallions, thinly sliced
1/8 teaspoon red-pepper flakes
1 teaspoon chopped, fresh thyme, plus more for garnish (optional)
1/4 teaspoon coarse salt
1 medium zucchini, halved lengthwise and sliced 1/2-inch thick
1 large celery stalk, diced
1 lime, halved

Preheat oven to 350 degrees. Toast almonds until crisp, lightly browned, and fragrant, about seven minutes. Remove from oven, and set aside. While almonds are toasting, place quinoa in a fine sieve, and rinse under cold running water until the water runs clear; drain well. In a medium saucepan, heat two teaspoons olive oil over medium heat. Add yellow pepper, garlic, scallions, and red-pepper flakes; cook until the pepper is crisp-tender, about five minutes. Stir in quinoa, thyme, one cup water, and one-fourth teaspoon salt. Bring to a boil, and then reduce to a simmer. Cover, and cook seven minutes.

Stir in zucchini; cover, and cook until quinoa is tender but not mushy, five to eight minutes longer. Remove the saucepan from heat. Stir in celery, almonds, and the remaining two teaspoons oil. Season with salt, and fluff with a fork. Cool to room temperature before packing into two containers and refrigerating. When you are ready to eat, squeeze lime over salad, if desired. Serve with an additional lime wedge and thyme, if desired.

Spicy Black-Bean Salad—Makes two servings
We are reintroducing lean proteins this week, and they will keep you satisfied and boost your energy.

Juice of 1 lime
2 tablespoons extra-virgin olive oil
1/4 teaspoon ground cumin
1 1/2 cups cooked black beans, drained
1/2 red bell pepper, stem and seeds removed, diced
1/4 red onion, diced
1 jalapeno, seeded and thinly sliced
1/4 cup fresh cilantro, chopped
2 cups baby spinach or arugula
Coarse salt

In a small bowl, whisk together lime juice, oil, and cumin. In a large bowl, combine beans, red pepper, onion, jalapeno, cilantro, and spinach. Drizzle with vinaigrette, and season with salt.

Kale, White Bean, and Potato Stew—Makes four servings

2 tablespoons extra-virgin olive oil, plus more for drizzling
1 onion, diced
1 stalk celery, sliced
1 carrot, peeled and diced
8 ounces Yukon Gold potatoes, scrubbed and cut into one-inch piece
Coarse salt and freshly ground pepper
1 bunch kale, stems removed, leaves torn into small pieces (4 cups)
1 (15-ounce) can navy beans, drained and rinsed
2 teaspoons red-wine vinegar

Heat oil in a medium saucepan over medium heat. Sauté onion, celery, and carrot until tender, about seven minutes. Add potatoes and four cups water. Season with salt and pepper. Bring to a boil; reduce to a simmer. Cook until potatoes are tender, about ten minutes. Mash half the contents of the pot until slightly thickened. Add kale and beans, and continue cooking until kale is tender, six to eight minutes more. Stir in vinegar, and adjust seasoning if necessary. Drizzle with oil before serving.

Roasted Beets with Edamame and Arugula –Makes (four servings)

3 medium golden beets
2 tablespoons, plus 1 teaspoon, olive oil, plus more for drizzling
1 cup frozen, shelled edamame, thawed
Coarse salt and pepper
1 tablespoon red-wine vinegar
3 cups baby arugula
1/2 cup fresh basil leaves

Heat oven to 425 degrees. Drizzle beets with olive oil, and roast in parchment-lined foil until tender, about one hour. Let cool, then peel and slice. On a baking sheet, toss edamame with one teaspoon olive oil; season with salt and pepper. Roast, shaking pan once, until golden, about twenty minutes.

In a small bowl, whisk vinegar and two tablespoons olive oil. In a medium bowl, combine arugula, basil, beets, and edamame. Toss with dressing, and season with salt and pepper.

Spaghetti with Sardines, Cauliflower, and Kale—Makes two servings

Sneak in more veggies by tossing in cauliflower and kale with your pasta.

3 tablespoons extra-virgin olive oil
2 halved and thinly sliced onions
Kosher salt and ground pepper
1 head cauliflower, cut into florets
1/2 teaspoon red-pepper flakes
1 bunch kale, torn into bite-size pieces
8 ounces whole-wheat spaghetti
1/2 tin sardines, broken into pieces
1 tablespoon lemon juice

Heat one tablespoon of oil in a large skillet over medium-high heat. Add onions; season with salt and pepper. Cook, stirring until golden, about eighteen minutes. (Reduce heat if onions become too dark.) Meanwhile, bring a large pot of salted water to a boil. Add cauliflower and red-pepper flakes, and cook for four minutes. Using a slotted spoon, transfer cauliflower to pan with onions.
Cook, stirring, until cauliflower is tender, about four minutes. Add kale to cauliflower. Cook, stirring, until kale is tender, about four minutes. Meanwhile, add spaghetti to boiling water; cook according to package instructions. Drain pasta, reserving one cup water; add to pan with cauliflower. Add just enough pasta water to create a sauce that coats the pasta. Remove from heat; stir in sardines, lemon juice, and two more tablespoons of oil. Season with salt and pepper. Serve immediately.

WEEK FOUR—DINNER

"If we eat wrongly, no doctors can cure us; if we eat rightly, no doctor is needed."—Victor G. Rocine

<u>Roasted Vegetables with Lentils</u> –Makes four servings
You can swap any veggie—brussels sprouts, turnips, or cabbage—into this warm salad. Just make sure you cut everything to about the same size for even roasting. Don't skip the celery leaves; they may seem delicate, but they pack a lot of flavor.

1/2 pound carrots, halved lengthwise
1 red onion, cut into one-inch wedges
1 small acorn squash, halved, seeds removed, cut into one-half-inch slices
5 tablespoons extra-virgin olive oil
Coarse salt and freshly ground pepper
1/2 cup dried French green lentils, rinsed
1 shallot, halved
4 teaspoons apple-cider vinegar
1 teaspoon Dijon mustard
1 stalk celery, thinly sliced, plus leaves

Heat oven to 425 degrees. On two baking sheets, arrange carrots, onion, and squash; drizzle with two tablespoons oil, and season with salt and pepper. Roast, turning once, until caramelized and tender, about thirty minutes. Meanwhile, place lentils and shallot in a medium saucepan, and cover with two inches of water. Bring to a boil, then simmer, covered, until lentils are tender, about twenty minutes. Drain; discard shallot. Season with salt and pepper. Combine vinegar and mustard. Pour remaining three tablespoons of oil in a slow, steady stream, whisking constantly. Toss lentils and celery with vinaigrette, and season with salt and pepper. Spoon over roasted vegetables. Garnish with celery leaves.

Roasted Shitakes and Pacific Cod—Makes four servings
Pacific cod makes a good environmental choice. Pacific halibut also works, but you may need to reduce the cooking time.

2 pounds shiitake mushrooms, stems removed, halved if large
4 tablespoons olive oil
4 sprigs fresh rosemary
4 pacific cod or halibut fillets (6 to 8 ounces each)
1 tablespoon fresh lemon juice
1 tablespoon Dijon mustard
Coarse salt and ground pepper

Preheat oven to 450 degrees. On a large rimmed baking sheet, toss mushrooms with two tablespoons olive oil and rosemary; season with salt and pepper. Roast until tender and browned, tossing occasionally, about fifteen minutes. Push mushrooms to the sides of the pan; place cod in center, and season with salt and pepper. Roast until opaque throughout, about ten minutes. Meanwhile, in a small bowl, whisk together remaining oil, lemon juice, mustard, and parsley; season with salt and pepper. Serve with cod.

Almond Chicken Soup with Sweet Potato, Collards, and Ginger—Makes two servings
Sweet potato and almond butter give this soup a creamy, decadent tex
4 cups chicken stock
1/2 yellow onion, diced
1 minced garlic clove

1 large sweet potato, peeled and diced (2 cups)
8 ounces boneless, skinless chicken breast, cut into one-inch pieces
1/2 cup smooth almond butter
1 cup collard leaves, coarsely chopped
2 tablespoons minced fresh ginger
Coarse salt and freshly ground black pepper
1 lime, cut into wedges

Combine the stock, onion, garlic, and sweet potato in a stockpot, and bring to a boil.

Reduce the heat to a simmer, and add the chicken. Then cover and simmer for twenty minutes.

In a small bowl, whisk together the almond butter and one-half cup of the soup mixture into a thick paste. Add the collard leaves and ginger to the soup, and bring to a boil. Then reduce the heat and simmer, covered, for five minutes. Stir in the almond-butter paste. Season with salt and pepper. Ladle the soup into bowls, and drizzle with lime juice.

Grilled Beef Skewers with Zucchini and Mint—Makes two servings

This meal is delicious any time of year and provides you with a healthy combination of whole grains, vegetables, and protein.

1 cup short-grain brown rice
2 cups water
3 scallions, thinly sliced
8 ounces grass-fed sirloin steak, trimmed, cut into one-and-one-half-inch cubes
2 zucchini, halved and cut into spears
Kosher salt and freshly ground black pepper
Extra-virgin olive oil, for drizzling
1/2 cup fresh mint leaves
1/2 teaspoon red-chili flakes
1 lime, cut into wedges, for serving

Bring rice and water to a boil. Reduce heat to a simmer and cover. Cook forty-five minutes, until tender. Let stand, covered, for five minutes. Fluff with a fork. Stir in scallions. Preheat a grill pan over medium-high heat. Thread beef on skewers. Season beef and zucchini with salt and pepper, and drizzle with oil. Grill, turning, until cooked through and blackened in parts, about seven minutes. Serve over rice. Top with mint leaves and red-chili flakes. Serve with lime wedges.

Shiitake Mushrooms and Brown Rice En Papillote—Makes two servings

Meaty shiitakes are one of the best foods to eat to support good health, boasting a special combination of antioxidants that boost immune function and lower oxidative stress in the body. Try substituting mushrooms for meat in meals; mushrooms slash calories and improve your well-being without leaving you hungry.

2 cups cooked brown rice
4 cups thinly sliced shiitake mushrooms
8 sprigs fresh thyme
Coarse salt and pepper
1/4 cup olive oil
1 cup fresh greens
Lemon wedges

Heat oven to 425 degrees. Cut four pieces of parchment paper, in twelve by sixteen rectangles. Divide brown rice equally among each parchment piece. Top with mushrooms and thyme. Season with salt and pepper, and drizzle with olive oil. Bake on a rimmed baking sheet until packet is puffed and mushrooms are cooked through, twenty minutes. Serve with a side of greens, and drizzle with lemon.

WEEKS ONE TO FOUR—SNACKS

Dried Fruit and Nut Bites
2 cups mixed dried fruit
2 cups raw mixed nuts and seeds
Dash of cinnamon
1/3 cup raw sesame seeds

In a food processor, pulse two cups mixed dried fruit, and transfer to a bowl. Pulse two cups raw mixed nuts and seeds until finely chopped. Add the nuts to the dried fruit, along with dash a of cinnamon and a pinch of sea salt. Knead together, and form one-inch balls. Roll each ball in one-third cup raw sesame seeds. Makes twenty bites.

Crispy Roasted Cauliflower
1 head of cauliflower
1 tablespoon olive oil
Red-pepper flakes

Heat oven to 425 degrees. On a rimmed baking sheet, drizzle cauliflower florets with one tablespoon olive oil. Season with salt. Roast, turning occasionally, about twenty minutes. Sprinkle with red-pepper flakes. Makes two cups.

<u>Cinnamon Poached Apples with Toasted Walnuts</u>
3 cups sugar-free apple juice
½ cinnamon stick
Fresh ginger
2 apples, cored and peeled and cut in half

Bring three cups apple juice, one-half cinnamon stick, and one inch fresh ginger, thinly sliced, to a boil. Add two cored, peeled, and halved apples. Simmer until tender, about eight minutes.
Remove and sprinkle with two tablespoons chopped, toasted walnuts. Serves two.

<u>Minty Pea or Edamame Dip</u>
Raw vegetables
3 cups peas or edamame
¼ cup fresh mint leaves
1 lemon
1 clove garlic
2 tablespoons EVOO
1 tablespoon tahini

Cook three cups frozen green peas (or edamame) in salted, boiling water until tender, about one minute. Transfer to an ice-water bath and drain. Pulse in food processor with one-fourth cup fresh mint leaves. Add and pulse again, the zest and juice of one lemon, one garlic clove, two tablespoons olive oil, and one tablespoon tahini. Season with salt and pepper; drizzle with oil. Serves four.

<u>Cranberry Pumpkin-Seed Trail Mix</u>
½ cup dried cranberries
½ cup almonds, chopped and toasted
½ cup pumpkin seeds, toasted

¼ cup walnuts, toasted
¼ cup raisins

Combine one-half cup dried cranberries, one-half cup chopped toasted almonds, one-half cup toasted pumpkin seeds, one-fourth cup toasted walnuts, and one-fourth cup raisins. Makes two cups of mix.

Pistachio-Stuffed Dates with Coconut
½ cup pistachios, shelled
16 dates, pitted
1 tablespoon unsweetened, shredded coconut

In a food processor, puree one-half cup shelled pistachios until a thick paste forms, about five minutes. Season with salt. Spoon mixture into sixteen pitted dates. Top with one tablespoon unsweetened, shredded coconut. Makes sixteen.

Other Snack Options

—One small apple (sliced) and one tablespoon of nut butter
—Air-popped popcorn with cinnamon and stevia or stove-popped using coconut oil
—Up to fifteen unsalted mixed nuts (almonds, walnuts, brazil nuts, or cashews)
—A tablespoon of nut butter on a celery stick
—One-fourth cup hummus or guacamole or salsa with celery sticks
—Dulse seaweed, either raw or toasted.
—One-fourth cup walnuts and one-half cup strawberries
—Toasted sunflower and pumpkin seeds mixed with raisins
—Boiled eggs

WEEK FIVE,—PHASE 3 (OPTIONAL)

This is the fasting phase, and it can be the most challenging but also the most productive. If you have completed phases one and two, you should be ready for a one- to-three-day fast. I have included a seven-day fast, which can be modified for one to three days. Following the fast, you will return to the phase two, weeks three and four of the program.

Fasting Choices

There are many fasting choices I would like to share with you. The lemonade fast is a powerful fast for the kidneys, digestive system, and liver. Lemon and lime are rich source of vitamins and minerals and help to reduce accumulation of toxins in the liver and stomach. Lemon also fights infections and builds up immunity. Another ingredient used in the lemonade fast, 100 percent pure maple syrup, supplies vitamins and minerals and enough sugar to sustain energy. It also curbs sweet cravings. The cayenne pepper in the recipe works as a stimulant to break up mucus and provide warmth to the digestive system. Ground ginger, working together with the cayenne pepper, speeds up the metabolism, helps to burn fat faster, and boosts circulation.

The Lemonade Fast Recipe

Combine eight cups pure water, the juice of four fresh lemons or limes, three tablespoons pure maple syrup, one-eighth teaspoon of cayenne pepper, and a pinch of ground ginger. Drink at room temperature. Make fresh daily. Drink six to twelve cups per day.

Preparation and the Fast

Days One and Two—Preparation Days
Begin each morning with the juice of half a lemon in eight ounces of water.
Take a brisk walk followed by stretching or yoga and deep breathing exercises.

Breakfast—Bowl of fresh fruit (no banana) or soft, nongluten grains
Lunch—Prepare a raw vegetable salad with lemon, garlic, and extra-virgin olive oil dressing for lunch (no avocados).
Dinner—Plate of steamed vegetables with lemon, garlic, and EVOO
For snacks in between meals, you can have a smoothie made with fresh vegetable juice or water, one tablespoon of ground flaxseed, one table-spoon of flaxseed oil, and green drink powder.

Days Three and Four (fasting days)
Breakfast—Drink ten ounces of lemonade mixture.
Take a walk followed by stretching or yoga and deep breathing exercises.
Throughout the day drink six to twelve glasses of the lemonade.

Day Five
Wake up—Drink ten ounces of the freshly made lemonade.
Break the fast with a piece of in-season, raw, organic fruit.

Lunch—Eat a salad with freshly grated cabbage, carrot, and beet tossed with fresh lemon juice. This will help the intestines get moving again.

Midday—Have a ten-ounce glass of fresh lemonade.

Dinner—Eat fresh vegetable salad or steamed vegetables with lemon, garlic, and EVOO.

Days Six and Seven

Wake up—Drink ten ounces of fresh lemonade.

Begin adding soft grains, vegetarian protein, and more cooked and raw vegetables into your meals.

Return to weeks three and four of the Mindful-Eating Program.

$\mathcal{H}$ANDBOOK

Do you experience any of these symptoms? Circle them now.

Headaches or migraines
Disturbed sleep
Watery or itchy eyes
Dark circles under your eyes
Itchy ears
Sneezing attacks
A chronic cough
A runny nose (but not a cold)
An itchy palate
A sore tongue
A furred tongue
Acne
Hives (nettle rash)
Other rashes
Hot flashes
Excessive sweating
Sweat with an unpleasant smell
Irregular heartbeat
Rapid heartbeat
Heartburn or indigestion
Nausea or vomiting
Diarrhea

Constipation
Bloated feeling
Belching
Mood swings
Passing excessive or offensive wind
Pain or stiffness in joints
Aching or painful muscles
Feeling shaky and weak
Binge eating
Binge drinking
Cravings for certain foods
Compulsive eating
Water retention
Urinary frequency
Feeling very tired in the morning
Being more tired than you would expect for your age
Feeling agitated without an obvious cause
Being restless and unable to settle
Having problems with memory
Feeling confused
Being unable to understand new information
Poor concentration
Clumsiness
Problems with your speech
Having difficulty making decisions
Unexplained feelings, such as anxiety or fear
Unprovoked anger, irritability, or aggressiveness
Depression
Sensitivity to light
Sensitivity to noise
ADD or hyperactivity
Arthritis (osteoarthritis or rheumatoid)
Bad breath
Mentally foggy (brain-fog feeling)

Chronic sinus problems
Difficulty losing weight
Eczema
IBS symptoms
PMS
Thyroid problems
Psoriasis
Craving breads/carbs
Craving sugar/alcohol
Burning urination
Athlete's foot/nail fungus
Vaginal or penile itching or burning
Symptoms worsen at night
Night sweats

How many symptoms do you have?_____

Current weight _____

Would you like your weight to be different? _____ If yes, what? _____

Starting measurements of waist?_____ Hips?_____ Thigh?_____

What is your goal? _____

MINDFUL, DAILY HELPFUL TIPS

These tips are repeated here as an easy-to-find tool to help you organize your day. They include everything you need for a successful mindful-eating program.

1. Set goals. Use the handbook attached in this book, or go buy a journal. Write down three to five goals and what it would mean to you to have complete them.

2. Prepare the people in your life. Explain your eating plan to people you normally eat meals with; they should know how important this program is to you so they can support you.

3. Invite a friend to join you. Even the most motivated person can derail. If you do this program with a partner, you can encourage each other.

4. Drink plenty of water. The water you drink flushes out the toxins in your system, keeps hunger at bay, and keeps you hydrated. Start every morning with warm water and a squeeze of lemon.

5. Space out your meals by eating every four to five hours rather than nonstop nibbling. Evenly spaced meals will keep your metabolism even.

6. Keep track of what, when, and where you eat and the amount of liquids you are consuming, as well as how you feel before, during, and after you eat. This will bring awareness and transform your relationship with food.

7. Stick to each week's menu. Different phases of the program offer different foods for a reason, so don't jump ahead.

8. Use Saturday and Sunday to do your shopping and to prep food for the week. Clean any fresh fruit and vegetables. Prepare dishes for the coming week. This may sound like a lot of time spent cooking, but it will save you time during the week.

9. Please note that most dinners are designed so you can use leftovers for lunch the next day.

10. If you are feeling full or in a rush, know that you can exchange a meal for a smoothie as long as you put in a scoop of protein powder and crushed flaxseeds or chia seeds.

11. Eat slowly, and chew your food well—about thirty times.

12. Hydrate. Drink one-half your body weight in ounces of water each day. (For example, if your weight is two hundred pounds, drink one hundred ounces of water.)

13. Try to go to bed at least thirty minutes earlier than you normally would.

Tips for Eating Out

1. Always choose wild fish over farm-raised fish.
2. Always choose grass-fed beef.
3. You can ask to switch all side dishes to two vegetables instead.
4. Always ask how the food is prepared.
5. Bring wheat-free pasta, and ask the chef to prepare it for you.
6. If you are not hungry, just order a few appetizers, or consider sharing an entrée.
7. Bring your own tea bag, and order a cup of hot water, or, instead of tea, order a cup of hot water with lemon.

Self-Care

Self-care is taking time out for you. Go ahead! Check your schedule. Make an appointment for yourself.

1. Have a gentle massage, reflexology, shiatsu, or any other type of bodywork to help increase circulation and aid in healing your body.
2. Dry brush your skin to help cleanse and stimulate your largest organ of elimination. Use a natural-bristle skin brush while your skin is dry, and begin with your feet, then move up toward your heart.
3. Deep-breathing exercises help to eliminate toxins through the lungs while calming and centering the mind and body.
4. Get outside for fifteen minutes, and allow your skin to absorb the sun.
5. Enjoy the amazing feeling of being alive, and be grateful for your life.

Mindful Eating "Good"-Food Choice List

<u>Fruits</u>
Apples
Blackberries
Blueberries
Boysenberries
Cherries
Cranberries
Pears
Pomegranates
Raspberries
Strawberries
Pineapple
Watermelon
Plums
Mangoes
Grapefruits

<u>Nuts and Seeds</u>
(unsalted, raw, dry roasted or nut butter)
Almonds

Pecans
Sesame
Hazelnuts
Brazil nuts
Pistachios
Walnuts
Pumpkin seeds

Protein
(organic, free range or wild)
Bison
Chicken
Cod
Halibut
Sole
Lamb
Wild salmon
Scallops
Turkey
Grass-fed Beef
Sardines
Shrimp

Beans
Black beans
Kidney beans
Lentils
Lima beans
Chickpeas
White beans

Vegetables
(fresh, raw, steamed, juiced, or roasted)
Arugula

Asparagus
Avocado
Beet greens
Bell peppers
Bok choy
Broccoli
Brussels sprouts
Cabbage
Cauliflower
Celery
Collard greens
Cucumber
Garlic
Green beans
Kale
Lettuce
Mustard greens
Onions
Snap peas
Snow peas
Spinach
Squash
Swiss char
Artichokes

Sweeteners
Stevia
Coconut sugar
Local honey

Karen Mayo
Certified Nutrition Health and Lifestyle Coach

Shoppers Guide to Pesticides In Produce
DIRTY DOZEN

APPLES
CELERY
CHERRY TOMATOES
CUCUMBERS
GRAPES
HOT PEPPERS

NECTARINES IMPORTED
PEACHES
POTATOES
SPINACH
STAWBERRIES
SWEET BELL PEPPERS

PLUS
COLLARDS & KALE
SUMMER SQUASH & ZUCCHINI*
*PESTICIDES OF SPECIAL CONCERN

Shoppers Guide to Pesticides In Produce
CLEAN FIFTEEN

ASPARAGUS
AVOCADO
CABBAGE
CANTALOUPE
CORN
EGGPLANT
GRAPEFRUIT

KIWI
MANGOS
MUSHROOMS
ONION
PAPAYAS
SWEET PEAS FROZEN
SWEET POTATOES

Week One—
Shopping List

<u>Fruits and Vegetables</u>
Grapefruits
Apples
Carrots
Lemons
Baby spinach
Beets
Cucumber
Pear
Celery
Romaine lettuce
Pineapple
Kale
Limes
Onion
Sweet Potatoes
Butternut squash
Portobello mushrooms
Red bell peppers
Broccoli
Red cabbage
Arugula

Watercress
Mixed greens

Fresh Herbs and Seeds
Fresh ginger
Fresh mint
Garlic
Fennel seeds
Sunflower seeds
Pumpkin seeds
Hemp seeds

Pantry
Dijon mustard
Apple-cider vinegar
Coconut oil
Capers

Spices
Turmeric
Cinnamon
Cardamom
Cumin
Curry powder

Protein
(organic, free range, or wild)
Striped bass fillets

Supplements
Probiotics (health food store)

WEEK ONE—DAY ONE

Write a positive goal that you would like to accomplish for yourself *personally* in the next three months. _____
_____
_____
_____
_____

Next write two action steps you need to take to make the goal happen. When will this goal be completed? What will accomplishing this goal mean to you? _____
_____
_____
_____
_____

Write a positive goal that you would like to accomplish for yourself *professionally* in the next three months. _____
_____
_____
_____
_____

Next write two action steps you need to take to make the goal happen. When will this goal be completed ? What will accomplishing this goal mean to you? _____
_____
_____

_____

_____

_____The positive affirmation of this week is about you, the physical human being. Your affirmation is "I am fearless." Repeat this as many times as you need to during the day to get through some of the tough moments of self-sabotage. Write the affirmation in your journal, and say it to yourself in the mirror. This is a really powerful tool. This affirmation is great when your mind is giving you excuses about why you don't have to do something. You can affirm that "I am fearless."_____

_____

_____

_____

_____Your mindful movement of the week will stimulate the elimination organs. Choose an exercise you love, and have fun doing it for thirty minutes for three days, to start. Walk, run, swim, do yoga, Pilates, tai-chi, bike, or dance. Turn up the music, and shake your groove thang, baby! Take the stairs instead of the elevator. Park your car in a parking spot farthest from the door. Be careful your first week; you don't want to break something. _____

_____

_____

_____

_____Your mindful meditation of the week is to be mindful about your relationship with your food. Visualize the care and love that was spent preparing the food. Think about how it feels going into your mouth, the textures, and how you enjoyed each nutritious bite._____

_____

_____

_____

_____

<u>Daily Checklist for Week One</u> _____

_____Stress foods eliminated (flour, refined sugar, dairy, coffee, black tea, and alcohol)

_____Food for the week is purchased.

_____Kitchen is organized for the week.

Wake up

_____Drink a cup of warm water with fresh lemon squeezed into it.

_____The mindful meditation of the week is to be mindful about your relationship with your food.

Breakfast

_____Probiotics supplements

_____Omega-3 fatty acid—either two to three tablespoons ground flaxseed or fish oil

_____Fiber

_____Breakfast choice from week one options_____

_____Drink eight ounces of water or herbal tea.

_____Use coconut milk or almond milk instead of cow's milk.

_____Record your drink and food intake in your handbook.

Snack

_____Drink more water. Try to drink sixteen ounces or more before lunch.

_____Ate from the approved snack list.

Lunch

_____Lunch choice from week one options _____

_____Drink eight ounces more of water.

_____Get outside for at least ten minutes to get some fresh air, or take a walk to visit with someone on a different floor at work.

_____Record your drink and food intake—what you had and any emotional triggers.

Midafternoon Snack

_____Eat from the approved snack list.

_____Drink sixteen ounces more of water before dinner.

Dinner

_____Dinner choices from week one options_____

_____Drink eight ounces of water after dinner.

Bedtime

_____You will want to go to bed earlier during this program. Give your body more rest and the healing time it needs.

_____The mindful meditation of the week is to be mindful about your relationship with your food.

_____Journal Exercise—Each night before bed, take some time to reflect over your day. Create intentions for the next day. At the week's end, you may want to journal about what your greatest accomplishment for the week was, biggest challenge you had this week, what your main health concern is this week. Did you experience self-sabotage this week, and, if so, how did you silence your mind? _____

_____

_____

_____

_____

_____

_____

_____

_____

_____

_____

_____

_____

_____

_____

_____

_____

_____

_____

Week One—Day Two

Write a positive goal that you would like to accomplish for yourself *personally* in the next three months._____

_____

_____

_____

Next write two action steps you need to take to make the goal happen. When will this goal be completed? What is will accomplishing this goal mean to you?_____

_____

_____

_____

_____

Write a positive goal that you would like to accomplish for yourself *professionally* in the next three months._____

_____

_____

_____

_____

Next write two action steps you need to take to make the goal happen. When will this goal be completed? What will accomplishing this goal mean to you?_____

_____

_____

_____

_____

_____The positive affirmation of this week is about you, the physical human being. Your affirmation is "I am fearless." Repeat this as many times as you need to during the day to get through some of the tough moments of self-sabotage. Write the affirmation in your journal, and say it to yourself in the mirror. This is a really powerful tool. This affirmation is great when your mind is giving you excuses about why you don't have to do something. You can affirm that "I am fear less." _____

_____

_____

_____

_____Your mindful movement of the week will stimulate the elimination organs. Choose an exercise you love, and have fun doing it for thirty minutes for three days, to start. Walk, run, swim, do yoga, Pilates, tai-chi, bike, or dance. Turn up the music and shake your groove thang, baby! Take the stairs instead of the elevator. Park your car in a parking spot farthest from the door. Be careful your first week; you don't want to break something.

_____Your mindful meditation of the week is to be mindful about your relationship with your food. Visualize the care and love that was spent preparing the food. Think about how it feels going into your mouth, the textures, and how you enjoyed each nutritious bite._____

_____

_____

_____

Daily Checklist for Week One _____

_____Stress foods eliminated (flour, refined sugar, dairy, coffee, black tea, and alcohol)

_____Food for the week is purchased.

_____Kitchen is organized for the week.

Wake up

_____Drink a cup of warm water with fresh lemon squeezed into it.

_____The mindful meditation of the week is to be mindful about your relationship with your food.

Breakfast

_____Probiotics supplements

_____Omega-3 fatty acid—either two to three tablespoons ground flaxseed or fish oil

_____Fiber

_____Breakfast choice from week one options_____

_____Drink eight ounces of water or herbal tea.

_____Use coconut milk or almond milk instead of cow's milk.

_____Record your drink and food intake in your handbook.

Snack

_____Drink more water. Try to drink sixteen ounces or more before lunch.

_____Ate from the approved snack list.

Lunch

_____Lunch choice from week one options_____

_____Drink eight ounces more of water.

_____Get outside for at least ten minutes to get some fresh air, or take a walk to visit with someone on a different floor at work.

_____Record your drink and food intake—what you had and any emotional triggers.

Midafternoon Snack

_____Eat from the approved snack list._____

_____Drink sixteen ounces more of water before dinner.

Dinner

_____Dinner choices from week one options_____

_____Drink eight ounces of water after dinner.

Bedtime

_____You will want to go to bed earlier during this program. Give your body more rest and the healing time it needs.

_____The mindful meditation of the week is to be mindful about your relationship with your food.

_____Journal Exercise—Each night before bed, take some time to reflect over your day. Create intentions for the next day. At the week's end, you may want to journal about what your greatest accomplishment for the week was, biggest challenge you had this week, what your main health concern is this week. Did you experience self-sabotage this week, and, if so, how did you silence your mind? _____

_____

_____

_____

_____

_____

_____

_____

_____

_____

_____

_____

_____

_____

_____

_____

_____

_____

_____

_____

_____

_____

_____

_____

_____

Week One—Day Three

Write a positive goal that you would like to accomplish for yourself *personally* in the next three months._____

_____

_____

_____

Next write two action steps you need to take to make the goal happen. When will this goal be completed? What will accomplishing this goal mean to you?_____

_____

_____

_____

_____

Write a positive goal that you would like to accomplish for yourself *professionally* in the next three months._____

_____

_____

_____

_____

Next write two action steps you need to take to make the goal happen. When will this goal be completed? What will accomplishing this goal mean to you? _____

_____

_____

_____

_____

_____

_____The positive affirmation of this week is about you, the physical human being. Your affirmation is "I am fearless." Repeat this as many times as you need to during the day to get through some of the tough moments of self-sabotage. Write the affirmation in your journal, and say it to yourself in the mirror. This is a really powerful tool. This affirmation is great when your mind is giving you excuses about why you don't have to do something. You can affirm that "I am fearless." __

_____
_____
_____

_____Your mindful movement of the week will stimulate the elimination organs. Choose an exercise you love, and have fun doing it for thirty minutes for three days, to start. Walk, run, swim, do yoga, Pilates, tai-chi, bike, or dance. Turn up the music, and shake your groove thang, baby! Take the stairs instead of the elevator. Park your car in a parking spot farthest from the door. Be careful your first week; you don't want to break something.

_____Your mindful meditation of the week is to be mindful about your relationship with your food. Visualize the care and love that was spent preparing the food. Think about how it feels going into your mouth, the textures, and how you enjoyed each nutritious bite. _____

_____
_____
_____

Daily Checklist for Week One
_____Stress foods eliminated (flour, refined sugar, dairy, coffee, black tea, and alcohol)
_____Food for the week is purchased.
_____Kitchen is organized for the week.

Wake up
_____Drink a cup of warm water with fresh lemon squeezed into it.
_____The mindful meditation of the week is to be mindful about your relationship with your food.
Breakfast
_____Probiotics supplements

_____Omega-3 fatty acid—either two to three tablespoons ground flaxseed or fish oil

_____Fiber

_____Breakfast choice from week one options_____

_____Drink eight ounces of water or herbal tea.

_____Use coconut milk or almond milk instead of cow's milk.

_____Record your drink and food intake in your handbook.

Snack

_____Drink more water. Try to drink sixteen ounces or more before lunch.

_____Ate from the approved snack list._____

Lunch

_____Lunch choice from week one options_____

_____Drink eight ounces more of water.

_____Get outside for at least ten minutes to get some fresh air, or take a walk to visit with someone on a different floor at work.

_____Record your drink and food intake—what you had and any emotional triggers.

Midafternoon Snack

_____Eat from the approved snack list.

_____Drink sixteen ounces more of water before dinner.

Dinner

_____Dinner choices from week one options._____

_____Drink eight ounces of water after dinner.

Bedtime

_____You will want to go to bed earlier during this program. Give your body more rest and the healing time it needs.

_____The mindful meditation of the week is to be mindful about your relationship with your food.

_____Journal Exercise—Each night before bed, take some time to reflect over your day. Create intentions for the next day. At the week's end, you may want to journal about what your greatest accomplishment for the week was, biggest challenge you had this week, what your main health concern is this week. Did you experience self-sabotage this week, and, if so, how did you silence your mind? _____

_____

_____

_____

_____

_____

_____

_____

_____

_____

_____

_____

_____

_____

_____

_____

_____

_____

_____

_____

_____

_____

_____

_____

_____

_____

_____

_____

_____

_____

Week One—Day Four

Write a positive goal that you would like to accomplish for yourself *personally* in the next three months._____
_____
_____
_____

_____Next write two action steps you need to take to make the goal happen. When will this goal be completed? What will accomplishing this goal mean to you?_____
_____
_____
_____
_____

Write a positive goal that you would like to accomplish for yourself *professionally* in the next three months. _____
_____
_____
_____

_____Next write two action steps you need to take to make the goal happen. When will this goal be completed? What will accomplishing this goal mean to you?_____
_____
_____
_____

_____The positive affirmation of this week is about you, the physical human being. Your affirmation is "I am fearless." Repeat this as many times as you need to during the day to get through some of the tough moments of self-sabotage. Write the affirmation in your journal, and say it to yourself in the mirror. This is a really powerful tool. This affirmation is great when your mind is giving you excuses about why you don't have to do something. You can affirm that "I am fearless." __

_____

_____

_____

_____Your mindful movement of the week will stimulate the elimination organs. Choose an exercise you love, and have fun doing it for thirty minutes for three days, to start. Walk, run, swim, do yoga, Pilates, tai-chi, bike, or dance. Turn up the music, and shake your groove thang, baby! Take the stairs instead of the elevator. Park your car in a parking spot farthest from the door. Be careful your first week; you don't want to break something.

_____Your mindful meditation of the week is to be mindful about your relationship with your food. Visualize the care and love that was spent preparing the food. Think about how it feels going into your mouth, the textures, and how you enjoyed each nutritious bite. _____

_____

_____

Daily Checklist for Week One
_____Stress foods eliminated (flour, refined sugar, dairy, coffee, black tea, and alcohol)
_____Food for the week is purchased.
_____Kitchen is organized for the week.

Wake up
_____Drink a cup of warm water with fresh lemon squeezed into it.
_____The mindful meditation of the week is to be mindful about your relationship with your food.
Breakfast
_____Probiotics supplements

_____Omega-3 fatty acid—either two to three tablespoons ground flaxseed or fish oil

_____Fiber

_____Breakfast choice from week one options_____

_____Drink eight ounces of water or herbal tea.

_____Use coconut milk or almond milk instead of cow's milk.

_____Record your drink and food intake in your handbook. _____

_____

Snack

_____Drink more water. Try to drink sixteen ounces or more before lunch.

_____Ate from the approved snack list.

Lunch

_____Lunch choice from week one options_____

_____Drink eight ounces more of water.

_____Get outside for at least ten minutes to get some fresh air, or take a walk to visit with someone on a different floor at work.

_____Record your drink and food intake—what you had and any emotional triggers._____

_____

Midafternoon Snack

_____Eat from the approved snack list.

_____Drink sixteen ounces more of water before dinner.

Dinner

_____Dinner choices from week one options._____

_____Drink eight ounces of water after dinner.

Bedtime

_____You will want to go to bed earlier during this program. Give your body more rest and the healing time it needs.

_____The mindful meditation of the week is to be mindful about your relationship with your food.

_____Journal Exercise—Each night before bed, take some time to reflect over your day. Create intentions for the next day. At the week's end, you may want to journal about what your greatest accomplishment for the week was, biggest challenge you had this week, what your main health concern is this week. Did you experience self-sabotage this week, and, if so, how did you silence your mind?_____

Week One—Day Five

Write a positive goal that you would like to accomplish for yourself *personally* in the next three months._____

_____

_____

_____

Next write two action steps you need to take to make the goal happen. When will this goal be completed? What will accomplishing this goal mean to you?_____

_____

_____

_____

Write a positive goal that you would like to accomplish for yourself *professionally* in the next three months._____

_____

_____

_____

Next write two action steps you need to take to make the goal happen. When will this goal be completed? What will accomplishing this goal mean to you?_____

_____

_____

_____

_____The positive affirmation of this week is about you, the physical human being. Your affirmation is "I am fearless." Repeat this as many times as you need to during the day to get through some of the tough moments of self-sabotage. Write the affirmation in your journal, and say it to yourself in the mirror. This is a really powerful tool. This affirmation is great when your mind is giving you excuses about why you don't have to do something. You can affirm that "I am fearless."_____

_____

_____

_____Your mindful movement of the week will stimulate the elimination organs. Choose an exercise you love, and have fun doing it for thirty minutes for three days, to start. Walk, run, swim, do yoga, Pilates, tai-chi, bike, or dance. Turn up the music, and shake your groove thang, baby! Take the stairs instead of the elevator. Park your car in a parking spot farthest from the door. Be careful your first week; you don't want to break something.

_____Your mindful meditation of the week is to be mindful about your relationship with your food. Visualize the care and love that was spent preparing the food. Think about how it feels going into your mouth, the textures, and how you enjoyed each nutritious bite._____

_____

_____

<u>Daily Checklist for Week One</u>

_____Stress foods eliminated (flour, refined sugar, dairy, coffee, black tea, and alcohol)

_____Food for the week is purchased.

_____Kitchen is organized for the week.

Wake up

_____Drink a cup of warm water with fresh lemon squeezed into it.

_____The mindful meditation of the week is to be mindful about your relationship with your food.

Breakfast

_____Probiotics supplements

_____Omega-3 fatty acid—either two to three tablespoons ground flaxseed or fish oil

_____Fiber

_____Breakfast choice from week one options_____

_____Drink eight ounces of water or herbal tea.

_____Use coconut milk or almond milk instead of cow's milk.

_____Record your drink and food intake in your handbook. _____

Snack

_____Drink more water. Try to drink sixteen ounces or more before lunch.

_____Ate from the approved snack list.

Lunch

_____Lunch choice from week one options_____

_____Drink eight ounces more of water.

_____Get outside for at least ten minutes to get some fresh air, or take a walk to visit with someone on a different floor at work.

_____Record your drink and food intake—what you had and any emotional triggers._____

Midafternoon Snack

_____Eat from the approved snack list._____

_____Drink sixteen ounces more of water before dinner.

Dinner

_____Dinner choices from week one options_____

_____Drink eight ounces of water after dinner.

Bedtime

_____You will want to go to bed earlier during this program. Give your body more rest and the healing time it needs.

_____The mindful meditation of the week is to be mindful about your relationship with your food.

_____Journal Exercise—Each night before bed, take some time to reflect over your day. Create intentions for the next day. At the week's end, you may want to journal about what your greatest accomplishment for the week was, biggest challenge you had this week, what your main health concern is this week. Did you experience self-sabotage this week, and, if so, how did you silence your mind? _____

_____

_____

_____

_____

_____

_____

_____

_____

_____

_____

_____

_____

_____

_____

_____

_____

_____

_____

_____

_____

_____

_____

_____

_____

_____

_____

_____

_____

_____

_____

_____

_____

_____

_____

Week One—Day Six

Write a positive goal that you would like to accomplish for yourself *personally* in the next three months._____
_____
_____
_____

Next write two action steps you need to take to make the goal happen. When will this goal be completed? What will accomplishing this goal mean to you?_____
_____
_____
_____

Write a positive goal that you would like to accomplish for yourself *professionally* in the next three months._____
_____
_____
_____

Next write two action steps you need to take to make the goal happen. When will this goal be completed? What will accomplishing this goal mean to you?_____
_____
_____
_____

_____The positive affirmation of this week is about you, the physical human being. Your affirmation is "I am fearless." Repeat this as many times as you need to during the day to get through some of the tough moments of self-sabotage. Write the affirmation in your journal, and say it to yourself in the mirror. This is a really powerful tool. This affirmation is great when your mind is giving you excuses about why you don't have to do something. You can affirm that "I am fearless."_____
_____
_____

_____Your mindful movement of the week will stimulate the elimination organs. Choose an exercise you love, and have fun doing it for thirty minutes for three days, to start. Walk, run, swim, do yoga, Pilates, tai-chi, bike, or dance. Turn up the music, and shake your groove thang, baby! Take the stairs instead of the elevator. Park your car in a parking spot farthest from the door. Be careful your first week; you don't want to break something.

_____Your mindful meditation of the week is to be mindful about your relationship with your food. Visualize the care and love that was spent preparing the food. Think about how it feels going into your mouth, the textures, and how you enjoyed each nutritious bite._____

_____

_____

_____

Daily Checklist for Week One
_____Stress foods eliminated (flour, refined sugar, dairy, coffee, black tea, and alcohol)
_____Food for the week is purchased.
_____Kitchen is organized for the week.
Wake up
_____Drink a cup of warm water with fresh lemon squeezed into it.
_____The mindful meditation of the week is to be mindful about your relationship with your food.
Breakfast
_____Probiotics supplements
_____Omega-3 fatty acid—either two to three tablespoons ground flaxseed or fish oil
_____Fiber
_____Breakfast choice from week one options_____
_____Drink eight ounces of water or herbal tea.
_____Use coconut milk or almond milk instead of cow's milk.

_____Record your drink and food intake in your handbook. _____

_____

_____

Snack

_____Drink more water. Try to drink sixteen ounces or more before lunch.

_____Ate from the approved snack list.

Lunch

_____Lunch choice from week one options_____

_____Drink eight ounces more of water.

_____Get outside for at least ten minutes to get some fresh air, or take a walk to visit with someone on a different floor at work.

_____Record your drink and food intake—what you had and any emotional triggers.

Midafternoon Snack

_____Eat from the approved snack list._____

_____Drink sixteen ounces more of water before dinner.

Dinner

_____Dinner choices from week one options_____

_____Drink eight ounces of water after dinner.

Bedtime

_____You will want to go to bed earlier during this program. Give your body more rest and the healing time it needs.

_____The mindful meditation of the week is to be mindful about your relationship with your food.

_____Journal Exercise—Each night before bed, take some time to reflect over your day. Create intentions for the next day. At the week's end, you may want to journal about what your greatest accomplishment for the week was, biggest challenge you had this week, what your main health concern is this week. Did you experience self-sabotage this week, and, if so, how did you silence your mind?_____

_____

_____

Week One—Day Seven

Write a positive goal that you would like to accomplish for yourself *personally* in the next three months._____

_____

_____

_____

Next write two action steps you need to take to make the goal happen. When will this goal be completed? What will accomplishing this goal mean to you?_____

_____

_____

_____

Write a positive goal that you would like to accomplish for yourself *professionally* in the next three months._____

_____

_____

_____

Next write two action steps you need to take to make the goal happen. When will this goal be completed? What will accomplishing this goal mean to you?_____

_____

_____

_____

_____The positive affirmation of this week is about you, the physical human being. Your affirmation is "I am fearless." Repeat this as many times as you need to during the day to get through some of the tough moments of self-sabotage. Write the affirmation in your journal, and say it to yourself in the mirror. This is a really powerful tool. This affirmation is great when your mind is giving you excuses about why you don't have to do something. You can affirm that "I am fearless."_____

_____

_____

_____Your mindful movement of the week will stimulate the elimination organs. Choose an exercise you love, and have fun doing it for thirty minutes for three days, to start. Walk, run, swim, do yoga, Pilates, tai-chi, bike, or dance. Turn up the music, and shake your groove thang, baby! Take the stairs instead of the elevator. Park your car in a parking spot farthest from the door. Be careful your first week; you don't want to break something.

_____Your mindful meditation of the week is to be mindful about your relationship with your food. Visualize the care and love that was spent preparing the food. Think about how it feels going into your mouth, the textures, and how you enjoyed each nutritious bite._____

_____

_____

Daily Checklist—Week One
_____Stress foods eliminated (flour, refined sugar, dairy, coffee, black tea, and alcohol)
_____Food for the week is purchased.
_____Kitchen is organized for the week.
Wake up
_____Drink a cup of warm water with fresh lemon squeezed into it.
_____The mindful meditation of the week is to be mindful about your relationship with your food.
Breakfast
_____Probiotics supplements
_____Omega-3 fatty acid—either two to three tablespoons ground flaxseed or fish oil
_____Fiber
_____Breakfast choice from week one options_____
_____Drink eight ounces of water or herbal tea.
_____Use coconut milk or almond milk instead of cow's milk.
_____Record your drink and food intake in your handbook.

Snack

_____Drink more water. Try to drink sixteen ounces or more before lunch.

_____Ate from the approved snack list._____

Lunch

_____Lunch choice from week one options_____

_____Drink eight ounces more of water.

_____Get outside for at least ten minutes to get some fresh air, or take a walk to visit with someone on a different floor at work.

_____Record your drink and food intake—what you had and any emotional triggers.

Midafternoon Snack

_____Eat from the approved snack list.

_____Drink sixteen ounces more of water before dinner.

Dinner

_____Dinner choices from week one options_____

_____Drink eight ounces of water after dinner.

Bedtime

_____You will want to go to bed earlier during this program. Give your body more rest and the healing time it needs.

_____The mindful meditation of the week is to be mindful about your relationship with your food.

_____Journal Exercise—Each night before bed, take some time to reflect over your day. Create intentions for the next day. At the week's end, you may want to journal about what your greatest accomplishment for the week was, biggest challenge you had this week, what your main health concern is this week. Did you experience self-sabotage this week, and, if so, how did you silence your mind?_____

_____

_____

_____

_____

_____

_____

_____

_____

_____

_____

_____

_____

_____

_____

_____

_____

_____

_____

If you don't feel great, and you do not have lots of energy after week one, you may need to repeat week one. That's all right; everyone is different. If this is the case for you, just repeat week one and then move on to week two.

Current weight? _____

Measurements of waist? _____ Hips? _____ Thigh? _____

Shopping List— Week Two

<u>Fruits and Vegetables</u>
Banana
Yellow onion
Celery
Carrots
Sweet potatoes
Oranges
Broccoli
Scallions
Lemons
Tomatoes
Turnip
Large leek
Rutabaga
Parsnips
Brussels sprouts
Avocado
Red onion
Bok choy
Butternut squash
Kale
Swiss char

Pomegranate
Watercress

Nuts, Seeds, and Fresh Herbs
(unsalted nuts, raw, dry roasted, or nut butter)
Flaxseed meal
Garlic
Fresh parsley
Pine nuts
Quinoa
Fresh chives
Lemongrass
Fresh cilantro
Fresh tarragon
Chickpeas
Toasted almonds or pecans
Walnuts

Protein
(organic, free range or wild)
Sardines
Two four-ounce wild salmon fillets

Beans
Dried red lentils
Cannellini beans

Pantry
Oat flour
Unsweetened shredded coconut
Baking powder
Vanilla extract
Dijon mustard
Honey

Capers
Sesame oil
Coconut oil
Extra-virgin olive oil
Red-wine vinegar
Balsamic vinegar
Apple-cider vinegar
Coconut milk
Almond milk
Orange juice

Week Two—Day One

Revisit your personal, positive goal._____

_____

_____

_____

Revisit your professional, positive goal._____

_____

_____

_____

_____The positive affirmation of the week concerns your relation-
ships. Finish this statement; "I am grateful for_____" and list reasons
why you are grateful for this person. Being grateful is a very positive
vibration that makes you feel good. Repeat the affirmation from last
week as well. Repeat affirmations as necessary. You can change your
grateful affirmations every day this week; you may have many reasons to
be grateful._____

_____

_____

_____

_____For your mindful movement of the week, it's time to increase
the amount of exercise you are doing to thirty minutes of exercise five
days this week; add in ten minutes of stretching before and after each
exercise period. Turn on the music, get up, and dance!_____

_____

_____

_____Your mindful meditation of the week is to be mindful of your
breathing. Sit cross-legged, with your back straight and your eyes closed,
on a cushion or on a chair. Pay attention to either the movement of your
abdomen as you breathing in and out or on the awareness of the breath

as it goes in and out of your nostrils. Put your right hand on your heart and your left hand on your abdomen. The point isn't to completely clear your mind of thought; the point is to be aware of your thoughts and learn to let them be. As thoughts come up, return your focus to the object of your meditation, such as the breathing. Close your eyes; take a deep breath that fills your abdomen all the way. Hold for a count of four, and slowly breathe out for a count of four. Do this four times. Open your eyes slowly, and you should have a different outlook on things.

_____

_____

_____

_____

Mindful Daily Checklist—Week Two

_____Following the Mindful-Eating Program completely.

_____Exercise daily (walk, run, swim, yoga, Pilates, tai-chi, bike, dance, walk up and down steps).

_____Food for the week is purchased.

_____Kitchen is organized for the week.

Wake up

_____Drink a cup of warm water with fresh lemon squeezed into it.

_____The mindful meditation of the week is to be mindful of your breathing while you sit cross-legged, with your back straight and your eyes closed, on a cushion or on a chair.

Breakfast

_____Probiotics supplements

_____Omega-3 fatty acids (either two to three tablespoons ground flaxseed or fish oil)

_____Fiber

_____Breakfast choice from week two or week one options_____

_____Drink eight ounces of water or herbal tea.

_____Use coconut milk or almond milk instead of cow's milk.

_____Record your drink and food intake in your handbook.

Snack

_____Drink more water. Try to drink sixteen ounces more before lunch.

_____Eat from the approved snack list._____

Lunch

_____Lunch choice from week two or week one options_____

_____Drink eight more ounces of water.

_____Get outside for at least ten minutes to get some fresh air, or take a walk to visit someone on the different floor at work.

_____Record your drink and food intake in your handbook.

Midafternoon Snack

_____Eat from the approved snack list. _____

_____Drink sixteen more ounces of water before dinner.

Dinner:

_____Dinner choices from week two or week one options._____

_____Drink eight more ounces of water after dinner.

_____Record your drink and food intake in your handbook.

Bedtime

_____Your mindful meditation of the week is to be mindful of your breathing. Sit cross-legged, with your back straight and your eyes closed, on a cushion or on a chair. Pay attention to either the movement of your abdomen as you breathing in and out or on the awareness of the breath as it goes in and out of your nostrils. Put your right hand on your heart and your left hand on your abdomen. The point isn't to completely clear your mind of thought; the point is to be aware of your thoughts and learn to let them be. As thoughts come up, return your focus to the object of your meditation, such as the breathing. Close your eyes; take a deep breath that fills your abdomen all the way. Hold for a count of four, and slowly breathe out for a count of four. Do this four times. Open your eyes slowly, and you should have a different outlook on things._____

_____

_____

_____

_____The mindful journal of the week is to write your affirmations of the week and your reasons why. At the week's end, journal about your greatest accomplishment for the week, the biggest challenge you had this week, and what are your main health concerns are this week. Did you experience self-sabotage this week? If so how did you silence your mind?_____

_____

_____

_____

_____

_____

_____

_____

_____

_____

_____

_____

_____

_____

_____

_____

_____

_____

Week Two—Day Two

Revisit your personal, positive goals._____

_____

_____

_____

_____

Revisit your professional, positive goals._____

_____

_____

_____

_____The positive affirmation of the week concerns your relation-ships. Finish this statement; "I am grateful for _____" and list reasons why you are grateful for this person. Being grateful is a very positive vibration that makes you feel good. Repeat the affirmation from last week as well. Repeat affirmations as necessary. You can change your grateful affirmations every day this week; you may have many reasons to be grateful._____

_____

_____

_____For your mindful movement of the week, it's time to increase the amount of exercise you are doing to thirty minutes of exercise five days this week; add in ten minutes of stretching before and after each exercise period. Turn on the music, get up, and dance!_____

_____

_____

_____

_____Your mindful meditation of the week is to be mindful of your breathing. Sit cross-legged, with your back straight and your eyes

closed, on a cushion or on a chair. Pay attention to either the movement of your abdomen as you breathing in and out or on the awareness of the breath as it goes in and out of your nostrils. Put your right hand on your heart and your left hand on your abdomen. The point isn't to completely clear your mind of thought; the point is to be aware of your thoughts and learn to let them be. As thoughts come up, return your focus to the object of your meditation, such as the breathing. Close your eyes; take a deep breath that fills your abdomen all the way. Hold for a count of four, and slowly breathe out for a count of four. Do this four times. Open your eyes slowly, and you should have a different outlook on things. _____

_____

_____

_____

_____

Mindful Daily Checklist—Week Two

_____Following the Mindful-Eating Program completely.

_____Exercise daily (walk, run, swim, yoga, Pilates, tai-chi, bike, dance, walk up and down steps).

_____Food for the week is purchased.

_____Kitchen is organized for the week.

Wake up

_____Drink a cup of warm water with fresh lemon squeezed into it.

_____The mindful meditation of the week is to be mindful of your breathing while you sit cross-legged, with your back straight and your eyes closed, on a cushion or on a chair.

Breakfast

_____Probiotics supplements

_____Omega-3 fatty acids (either two to three tablespoons ground flaxseed or fish oil)

_____Fiber

_____Breakfast choice from week two or week one options_____
_____Drink eight ounces of water or herbal tea.
_____Use coconut milk or almond milk instead of cow's milk.
_____Record your drink and food intake in your handbook._____

Snack
_____Drink more water. Try to drink sixteen ounces more before lunch.
_____Eat from the approved snack list._____

Lunch
_____Lunch choice from week two or week one options_____
_____Drink eight more ounces of water.
_____Get outside for at least ten minutes to get some fresh air, or take a walk to visit someone on the different floor at work.
_____Record your drink and food intake in your handbook._____

Midafternoon Snack
_____Eat from the approved snack list._____
_____Drink sixteen more ounces of water before dinner.

Dinner:
_____Dinner choices from week two or week one options_____
_____Drink eight more ounces of water after dinner.
____Record your drink and food intake in your handbook._____

Bedtime

_____Your mindful meditation of the week is to be mindful of your breathing. Sit cross-legged, with your back straight and your eyes closed, on a cushion or on a chair. Pay attention to either the movement of your abdomen as you breathing in and out or on the awareness of the breath as it goes in and out of your nostrils. Put your right hand on your heart and your left hand on your abdomen. The point isn't to completely clear your mind of thought; the point is to be aware of your thoughts and learn to let them be. As thoughts come up, return your focus to the object of your meditation, such as the breathing. Close your eyes; take a deep breath that fills your abdomen all the way. Hold for a count of four, and slowly breathe out for a count of four. Do this four times. Open your eyes slowly, and you should have a different outlook on things. _____

_____

_____

_____

_____

_____The mindful journal of the week is to write your affirmations of the week and your reasons why. At the week's end, journal about your greatest accomplishment for the week, the biggest challenge you had this week, and what are your main health concerns are this week. Did you experience self-sabotage this week? If so how did you silence your mind?_____

_____

_____

_____

_____

_____

_____

_____

_____

_____

_____

_____

_____

_____

_____

Week Two—Day Three

Revisit your personal, positive goals._____
_____
_____
_____

Revisit your professional, positive goals._____
_____
_____
_____

_____The positive affirmation of the week concerns your relation-ships. Finish this statement; "I am grateful for _____" and list reasons why you are grateful for this person. Being grateful is a very positive vibration that makes you feel good. Repeat the affirmation from last week as well. Repeat affirmations as necessary. You can change your grateful affirmations every day this week; you may have many reasons to be grateful._____
_____
_____

_____For your mindful movement of the week, it's time to increase the amount of exercise you are doing to thirty minutes of exercise five days this week; add in ten minutes of stretching before and after each exercise period. Turn on the music, get up, and dance!_____
_____
_____

_____Your mindful meditation of the week is to be mindful of your breathing. Sit cross-legged, with your back straight and your eyes closed, on a cushion or on a chair. Pay attention to either the move-ment of your abdomen as you breathing in and out or on the aware-ness of the breath as it goes in and out of your nostrils. Put your right hand on your heart and your left hand on your abdomen. The point isn't to completely clear your mind of thought; the point is to be aware of your thoughts and learn to let them be. As thoughts come up, return your focus to the object of your meditation, such as the breathing. Close your eyes; take a deep breath that fills your abdomen all the way. Hold for a count of four, and slowly breathe out for a count of four. Do this four times. Open your eyes slowly, and you should have a different outlook on things._____

_____

_____

_____

Mindful Daily Checklist—Week Two

_____Following the Mindful-Eating Program completely.

_____Exercise daily (walk, run, swim, yoga, Pilates, tai-chi, bike, dance, walk up and down steps).

_____Food for the week is purchased.

_____Kitchen is organized for the week.

Wake up

_____Drink a cup of warm water with fresh lemon squeezed into it.

_____The mindful meditation of the week is to be mindful of your breathing while you sit cross-legged, with your back straight and your eyes closed, on a cushion or on a chair.

Breakfast

_____Probiotics supplements

_____Omega-3 fatty acids (either two to three tablespoons ground flaxseed or fish oil)

_____Fiber

_____Breakfast choice from week two or week one options_____

_____

_____Drink eight ounces of water or herbal tea.

_____Use coconut milk or almond milk instead of cow's milk.

_____Record your drink and food intake in your handbook._____

Snack

_____Drink more water. Try to drink sixteen ounces more before lunch.

_____Eat from the approved snack list._____

Lunch

_____Lunch choice from week two or week one options_____

_____Drink eight more ounces of water.

_____Get outside for at least ten minutes to get some fresh air, or take a walk to visit someone on the different floor at work.

_____Record your drink and food intake in your handbook._____

Midafternoon Snack

_____Eat from the approved snack list._____

_____Drink sixteen more ounces of water before dinner.

Dinner:

_____Dinner choices from week two or week one options_____

_____Drink eight more ounces of water after dinner.

_____Record your drink and food intake in your handbook._____

Bedtime

_____Your mindful meditation of the week is to be mindful of your breathing. Sit cross-legged, with your back straight and your eyes closed, on a cushion or on a chair. Pay attention to either the movement of your abdomen as you breathing in and out or on the awareness of the breath as it goes in and out of your nostrils. Put your right hand on your heart and your left hand on your abdomen. The point isn't to completely clear your mind of thought; the point is to be aware of your thoughts and learn to let them be. As thoughts come up, return your focus to the object of your meditation, such as the breathing. Close your eyes; take a deep breath that fills your abdomen all the way. Hold for a count of four, and slowly breathe out for a count of four. Do this four times. Open your eyes slowly, and you should have a different outlook on things. _____

_____

_____

_____

_____

_____The mindful journal of the week is to write your affirmations of the week and your reasons why. At the week's end, journal about your greatest accomplishment for the week, the biggest challenge you had this week, and what are your main health concerns are this week. Did you experience self-sabotage this week? If so how did you silence your mind?_____

_____

_____

_____

_____

_____

_____

_____

_____

_____

_____

_____

_____

Week Two—Day Four

Revisit your personal, positive goals._____

_____

_____

_____

Revisit your professional, positive goals.

_____

_____

_____

_____

_____The positive affirmation of the week concerns your relation-ships. Finish this statement; "I am grateful for _____" and list reasons why you are grateful for this person. Being grateful is a very positive vibration that makes you feel good. Repeat the affirmation from last week as well. Repeat affirmations as necessary. You can change your grateful affirmations every day this week; you may have many reasons to be grateful._____

_____

_____

_____For your mindful movement of the week, it's time to increase the amount of exercise you are doing to thirty minutes of exercise five days this week; add in ten minutes of stretching before and after each exercise period. Turn on the music, get up, and dance!_____

_____

_____

_____Your mindful meditation of the week is to be mindful of your breathing. Sit cross-legged, with your back straight and your eyes closed, on a cushion or on a chair. Pay attention to either the move-ment of your abdomen as you breathing in and out or on the awareness of the breath as it goes in and out of your nostrils. Put your right hand on your heart and your left hand on your abdomen. The point isn't to completely clear your mind of thought; the point is to be aware of your thoughts and learn to let them be. As thoughts come up, return your focus to the object of your meditation, such as the breathing. Close your eyes; take a deep breath that fills your abdomen all the way. Hold for a count of four, and slowly breathe out for a count of four. Do this four times. Open your eyes slowly, and you should have a different out-look on things. _____

_____

_____

_____

Mindful Daily Checklist for Week Two

_____Following the Mindful-Eating Program completely.

_____Exercise daily (walk, run, swim, yoga, Pilates, tai-chi, bike, dance, walk up and down steps).

_____Food for the week is purchased.

_____Kitchen is organized for the week.

Wake up

_____Drink a cup of warm water with fresh lemon squeezed into it.

_____The mindful meditation of the week is to be mindful of your breathing while you sit cross-legged, with your back straight and your eyes closed, on a cushion or on a chair.

Breakfast

_____Probiotics supplements

_____Omega-3 fatty acids (either two to three tablespoons ground flaxseed or fish oil)

_____Fiber

_____Breakfast choice from week two or week one options_____

_____

_____Drink eight ounces of water or herbal tea.

_____Use coconut milk or almond milk instead of cow's milk.

_____Record your drink and food intake in your handbook._____

Snack

_____Drink more water. Try to drink sixteen ounces more before lunch.

_____Eat from the approved snack list._____

Lunch

_____Lunch choice from week two or week one options_____

_____Drink eight more ounces of water.

_____Get outside for at least ten minutes to get some fresh air, or take a walk to visit someone on the different floor at work.

_____Record your drink and food intake in your handbook._____

Midafternoon Snack

_____Eat from the approved snack list._____

_____Drink sixteen more ounces of water before dinner.

Dinner:

_____Dinner choices from week two or week one options._____

_____Drink eight more ounces of water after dinner.

_____Record your drink and food intake in your handbook._____

Bedtime

_____Your mindful meditation of the week is to be mindful of your breathing. Sit cross-legged, with your back straight and your eyes closed, on a cushion or on a chair. Pay attention to either the movement of your abdomen as you breathing in and out or on the awareness of the breath as it goes in and out of your nostrils. Put your right hand on your heart and your left hand on your abdomen. The point isn't to completely clear your mind of thought; the point is to be aware of your thoughts and learn to let them be. As thoughts come up, return your focus to the object of your meditation, such as the breathing. Close your eyes; take a deep breath that fills your abdomen all the way. Hold for a count of four, and slowly breathe out for a count of four. Do this four times. Open your eyes slowly, and you should have a different outlook on things. _____

_____

_____

_____

_____The mindful journal of the week is to write your affirmations of the week and your reasons why. At the week's end, journal about your greatest accomplishment for the week, the biggest challenge you had this week, and what are your main health concerns are this week. Did you experience self-sabotage this week? If so how did you silence your mind? _____

_____

_____

_____

_____

_____

_____

_____

_____

_____

_____

_____

_____

_____

Week Two—Day Five

Revisit your personal, positive goals._____

_____

_____

_____

Revisit your professional, positive goals._____

_____

_____

_____

_____The positive affirmation of the week concerns your relationships. Finish this statement; "I am grateful for _____" and list reasons why you are grateful for this person. Being grateful is a very positive vibration that makes you feel good. Repeat the affirmation from last week as well. Repeat affirmations as necessary. You can change your grateful affirmations every day this week; you may have many reasons to be grateful._____

_____

_____

_____

_____For your mindful movement of the week, it's time to increase the amount of exercise you are doing to thirty minutes of exercise five days this week; add in ten minutes of stretching before and after each exercise period. Turn on the music, get up, and dance! _____

_____

_____

_____

_____Your mindful meditation of the week is to be mindful of your breathing. Sit cross-legged, with your back straight and your eyes closed, on a cushion or on a chair. Pay attention to either the movement of your abdomen as you breathing in and out or on the awareness of the breath as it goes in and out of your nostrils. Put your right hand on your heart and your left hand on your abdomen. The point isn't to completely clear your mind of thought; the point is to be aware of your thoughts and learn to let them be. As thoughts come up, return your focus to the object of your meditation, such as the breathing. Close your eyes; take a deep breath that fills your abdomen all the way. Hold for a count of four, and slowly breathe out for a count of four. Do this four times. Open your eyes slowly, and you should have a different outlook on things. _____

_____

_____

_____

Mindful Daily Checklist for Week Two
_____Following the Mindful-Eating Program completely.
_____Exercise daily (walk, run, swim, yoga, Pilates, tai-chi, bike, dance, walk up and down steps).
_____Food for the week is purchased.
_____Kitchen is organized for the week.

Wake up
_____Drink a cup of warm water with fresh lemon squeezed into it.
_____The mindful meditation of the week is to be mindful of your breathing while you sit cross-legged, with your back straight and your eyes closed, on a cushion or on a chair.

Breakfast
_____Probiotics supplements
_____Omega-3 fatty acids (either two to three tablespoons ground flaxseed or fish oil)
_____Fiber
_____Breakfast choice from week two or week one options _____

_____

_____Drink eight ounces of water or herbal tea.

_____Use coconut milk or almond milk instead of cow's milk.

_____Record your drink and food intake in your handbook. _____

Snack

_____Drink more water. Try to drink sixteen ounces more before lunch.

_____Eat from the approved snack list._____

Lunch

_____Lunch choice from week two or week one options_____

_____Drink eight more ounces of water.

_____Get outside for at least ten minutes to get some fresh air, or take a walk to visit someone on the different floor at work.

_____Record your drink and food intake in your handbook._____

Midafternoon Snack

_____Eat from the approved snack list._____

_____Drink sixteen more ounces of water before dinner.

Dinner:

_____Dinner choices from week two or week one options_____

_____Drink eight more ounces of water after dinner.

_____Record your drink and food intake in your handbook._____

Bedtime

_____ Your mindful meditation of the week is to be mindful of your breathing. Sit cross-legged, with your back straight and your eyes closed, on a cushion or on a chair. Pay attention to either the movement of your abdomen as you breathing in and out or on the awareness of the breath as it goes in and out of your nostrils. Put your right hand on your heart and your left hand on your abdomen. The point isn't to completely clear your mind of thought; the point is to be aware of your thoughts and learn to let them be. As thoughts come up, return your focus to the object of your meditation, such as the breathing. Close your eyes; take a deep breath that fills your abdomen all the way. Hold for a count of four, and slowly breathe out for a count of four. Do this four times. Open your eyes slowly, and you should have a different outlook on things._____

_____

_____

_____

_____

_____The mindful journal of the week is to write your affirmations of the week and your reasons why. At the week's end, journal about your greatest accomplishment for the week, the biggest challenge you had this week, and what are your main health concerns are this week. Did you experience self-sabotage this week? If so how did you silence your mind? _____

_____

_____

_____

_____

_____

_____

_____

_____

_____

_____

_____

Week Two—Day Six

Revisit your personal, positive goals._____
_____
_____
_____

Revisit your professional, positive goals. _____
_____
_____

_____The positive affirmation of the week concerns your relation-
ships. Finish this statement; "I am grateful for _____" and list reasons
why you are grateful for this person. Being grateful is a very positive
vibration that makes you feel good. Repeat the affirmation from last
week as well. Repeat affirmations as necessary. You can change your
grateful affirmations every day this week; you may have many reasons
to be grateful. _____
_____
_____
_____

_____For your mindful movement of the week, it's time to increase
the amount of exercise you are doing to thirty minutes of exercise five
days this week; add in ten minutes of stretching before and after each
exercise period. Turn on the music, get up, and dance! _____
_____
_____
_____

_____Your mindful meditation of the week is to be mindful of your
breathing. Sit cross-legged, with your back straight and your eyes
closed, on a cushion or on a chair. Pay attention to either the movement of your abdomen as you breathing in and out or on the awareness

of the breath as it goes in and out of your nostrils. Put your right hand on your heart and your left hand on your abdomen. The point isn't to completely clear your mind of thought; the point is to be aware of your thoughts and learn to let them be. As thoughts come up, return your focus to the object of your meditation, such as the breathing. Close your eyes; take a deep breath that fills your abdomen all the way. Hold for a count of four, and slowly breathe out for a count of four. Do this four times. Open your eyes slowly, and you should have a different outlook on things. _____

_____

_____

_____

_____

Mindful Daily Checklist for Week Two

_____Following the Mindful-Eating Program completely.

_____Exercise daily (walk, run, swim, yoga, Pilates, tai-chi, bike, dance, walk up and down steps).

_____Food for the week is purchased.

_____Kitchen is organized for the week.

Wake up

_____Drink a cup of warm water with fresh lemon squeezed into it.

_____The mindful meditation of the week is to be mindful of your breathing while you sit cross-legged, with your back straight and your eyes closed, on a cushion or on a chair.

Breakfast

_____Probiotics supplements

_____Omega-3 fatty acids (either two to three tablespoons ground flaxseed or fish oil)

_____Fiber

_____Breakfast choice from week two or week one options_____

_____

_____Drink eight ounces of water or herbal tea.

_____Use coconut milk or almond milk instead of cow's milk.

_____Record your drink and food intake in your handbook._____

Snack

_____Drink more water. Try to drink sixteen ounces more before lunch.

_____Eat from the approved snack list._____

Lunch

_____Lunch choice from week two or week one options_____

_____Drink eight more ounces of water.

_____Get outside for at least ten minutes to get some fresh air, or take a walk to visit someone on the different floor at work.

_____Record your drink and food intake in your handbook._____

Midafternoon Snack

_____Eat from the approved snack list._____

_____Drink sixteen more ounces of water before dinner.

Dinner:

_____Dinner choices from week two or week one options _____

_____Drink eight more ounces of water after dinner.

_____Record your drink and food intake in your handbook._____

Bedtime

_____Your mindful meditation of the week is to be mindful of your breathing. Sit cross-legged, with your back straight and your eyes

closed, on a cushion or on a chair. Pay attention to either the movement of your abdomen as you breathing in and out or on the awareness of the breath as it goes in and out of your nostrils. Put your right hand on your heart and your left hand on your abdomen. The point isn't to completely clear your mind of thought; the point is to be aware of your thoughts and learn to let them be. As thoughts come up, return your focus to the object of your meditation, such as the breathing. Close your eyes; take a deep breath that fills your abdomen all the way. Hold for a count of four, and slowly breathe out for a count of four. Do this four times. Open your eyes slowly, and you should have a different outlook on things. _____

_____
_____
_____
_____

_____The mindful journal of the week is to write your affirmations of the week and your reasons why. At the week's end, journal about your greatest accomplishment for the week, the biggest challenge you had this week, and what are your main health concerns are this week. Did you experience self-sabotage this week? If so how did you silence your mind? _____

_____
_____
_____
_____
_____
_____
_____
_____
_____
_____
_____
_____

Week Two—Day Seven

Revisit your personal, positive goals. _____

_____

_____

_____

Revisit your professional, positive goals._____

_____

_____

_____

_____The positive affirmation of the week concerns your relation-ships. Finish this statement; "I am grateful for _____" and list reasons why you are grateful for this person. Being grateful is a very positive vibration that makes you feel good. Repeat the affirmation from last week as well. Repeat affirmations as necessary. You can change your grateful affirmations every day this week; you may have many reasons to be grateful. _____

_____

_____

_____

_____For your mindful movement of the week, it's time to increase the amount of exercise you are doing to thirty minutes of exercise five days this week; add in ten minutes of stretching before and after each exercise period. Turn on the music, get up, and dance! _____

_____

_____

_____

_____Your mindful meditation of the week is to be mindful of your breathing. Sit cross-legged, with your back straight and your eyes closed, on a cushion or on a chair. Pay attention to either the movement of your abdomen as you breathing in and out or on the awareness of the breath as it goes in and out of your nostrils. Put your right hand on your heart and your left hand on your abdomen. The point isn't to completely clear your mind of thought; the point is to be aware of your thoughts and learn to let them be. As thoughts come up, return your focus to the object of your meditation, such as the breathing. Close your eyes; take a deep breath that fills your abdomen all the way. Hold for a count of four, and slowly breathe out for a count of four. Do this four times. Open your eyes slowly, and you should have a different outlook on things.

_____

_____

_____

_____

Mindful Daily Checklist for Week Two

_____Following the Mindful-Eating Program completely.

_____Exercise daily (walk, run, swim, yoga, Pilates, tai-chi, bike, dance, walk up and down steps).

_____Food for the week is purchased.

_____Kitchen is organized for the week.

Wake up

_____Drink a cup of warm water with fresh lemon squeezed into it.

_____The mindful meditation of the week is to be mindful of your breathing while you sit cross-legged, with your back straight and your eyes closed, on a cushion or on a chair.

Breakfast

_____Probiotics supplements

_____Omega-3 fatty acids (either two to three tablespoons ground flaxseed or fish oil)

_____Fiber

_____Breakfast choice from week two or week one options _____

_____

_____Drink eight ounces of water or herbal tea.

_____Use coconut milk or almond milk instead of cow's milk.

_____Record your drink and food intake in your handbook. _____

Snack

_____Drink more water. Try to drink sixteen ounces more before lunch.

_____Eat from the approved snack list._____

Lunch

_____Lunch choice from week two or week one options _____

_____Drink eight more ounces of water.

_____Get outside for at least ten minutes to get some fresh air, or take a walk to visit someone on the different floor at work.

_____Record your drink and food intake in your handbook._____

Midafternoon Snack

_____Eat from the approved snack list._____

_____Drink sixteen more ounces of water before dinner.

Dinner:

_____Dinner choices from week two or week one options_____

_____Drink eight more ounces of water after dinner.

_____Record your drink and food intake in your handbook. _____

Bedtime

_____Your mindful meditation of the week is to be mindful of your breathing. Sit cross-legged, with your back straight and your eyes

closed, on a cushion or on a chair. Pay attention to either the movement of your abdomen as you breathing in and out or on the awareness of the breath as it goes in and out of your nostrils. Put your right hand on your heart and your left hand on your abdomen. The point isn't to completely clear your mind of thought; the point is to be aware of your thoughts and learn to let them be. As thoughts come up, return your focus to the object of your meditation, such as the breathing. Close your eyes; take a deep breath that fills your abdomen all the way. Hold for a count of four, and slowly breathe out for a count of four. Do this four times. Open your eyes slowly, and you should have a different outlook on things.

_____

_____

_____

_____

_____The mindful journal of the week is to write your affirmations of the week and your reasons why. At the week's end, journal about your greatest accomplishment for the week, the biggest challenge you had this week, and what are your main health concerns are this week. Did you experience self-sabotage this week? If so how did you silence your mind? _____

_____

_____

_____

_____

_____

_____

_____

_____

_____

_____

_____

Current weight? _____

Measurements of waist? _____ Hips? _____ Thigh? _____

What is your goal? _____

Has it changed? _____

SHOPPING LIST— WEEK THREE

<u>Fruits and Vegetables</u>
Bananas
Scallions
Kale
Apples
Fresh berries
Red onion
Roasted red pepper
Onion
Acorn squash
Spinach
Red cabbage
Squash
Lemons
Red beets
Green leaf lettuce
Broccoli
Avocado
Lime

Nuts, Seeds, and Herbs
(unsalted nuts, raw, dry roasted, or nut butter)
Toasted sunflower seeds
Walnuts
Toasted almonds
Extra-virgin olive oil
Fresh basil
Fresh dill
Fresh parsley and chives
Fresh sage and thyme
Bay leaf
Paprika
Cumin
Garlic cloves

Protein
(organic, free range, or wild)
Eggs
Four wild salmon fillets (four ounces each)
Four cod fillets (four to six ounces each)

Beans
Black beans
Chickpeas

Pantry
Buckwheat flour
Baking powder
Honey
Unsweetened coconut flakes
Gluten-free rolled oats
Brown rice
Rice noodles
Corn tortillas
Quinoa

Week Three—Day One

Revisit your personal, positive goals. _____
_____
_____
_____

Revisit your professional, positive goals. _____
_____
_____
_____

_____Your positive affirmation of the week concerns your career or occupation The principle you will be putting into practice is "*a part of all I earn is mine to keep*". This principle is based on paying yourself first as you work toward accumulating wealth. Save at least 10 percent of what you earn each week, and put it into a separate account. When you are ready to celebrate you, this money will be there ready to use. This habit will help you develop a new, healthy mind-set. This is your third affirmation to remind yourself of every day. Keep writing the affirmations in your journal. _____
_____
_____
_____
_____
_____

_____The movement of the week will stimulate the elimination organs. This week's movement is thirty minutes of exercise for five days. Continue stretching for ten minutes before and after you exercise. Turn on the music, get up, and dance! Make an appointment for a massage, or get into a sauna this week._____
_____
_____
_____

_____The mindful meditation of the week is a visualization exercise. What do you envision the end result of this program looking like for you? How will the people in your life celebrate you? Do you just want to feel better in your clothes? Be really clear about your goals; visualize every detail. How will you feel? Dig deeper and really examine your feelings. What do you want six months from now to look like for you? How about one year from now?

_____

_____

_____

_____

_____

_____

Daily Checklist—Week Three

_____Food for the week is purchased.

_____Stay focused on the Mindful-Eating Program.

_____Kitchen is organized for the week.

Wake up

_____Drink a cup of warm water with fresh lemon squeezed into it.

_____Do your mindful meditation of the week.

Breakfast

_____Probiotics supplements

_____Omega-3 fatty acid (either two to three tablespoons of ground flaxseed or fish oil)

_____Fiber

_____Breakfast choice from week three options_____

_____

_____Drink eight ounces of water or herbal tea.

_____Use coconut milk or almond milk instead of cow's milk.

_____Record your drink and food intake in your handbook._____

_____

Snack

_____Drink more water; try to drink sixteen ounces more before lunch.

_____Eat from the approved snack list._____

Lunch

_____Lunch choice from week three options_____

_____

_____Drink eight ounces more of water.

_____Get outside for at least ten minutes to get some fresh air, or take a walk to visit with someone on a different floor of your office.

_____Record your drink and food intake in your handbook._____

_____

Midafternoon Snack

_____Eat from the approved snack list._____

_____Drink sixteen ounces of water, or more, before dinner.

Dinner

_____Dinner choices from week three options _____

_____

_____Drink eight ounces of water after dinner

Bedtime

_____ The mindful meditation of the week is a visualization exercise. What do you envision the end result of this program looking like for you? How will the people in your life celebrate you? Do you just want to feel better in your clothes? Be really clear about your goals; visualize every detail. How will you feel? Dig deeper and really examine your feelings. What do you want six months from now to look like for you? How about one year from now?_____

_____

_____

_____

_____

_____

_____The journal exercise of the week is to write down your visualization exercise. Remember to be very specific. At the week's end, journal about your greatest accomplishment of the week, the biggest challenge you had this week, and what your main health concern is at this time. _____

_____

_____

_____

_____

_____

_____

_____

_____

_____

_____

_____

_____

_____

_____

_____

_____

_____

_____

_____

_____

_____

_____

_____

_____

_____

_____

_____

Week Three—Day Two

Revisit your personal, positive goals._____
_____
_____
_____
_____

Revisit your professional, positive goals. _____
_____
_____
_____
_____

_____Your positive affirmation of the week concerns your career or occupation The principle you will be putting into practice is "*a part of all I earn is mine to keep*". This principle is based on paying yourself first as you work toward accumulating wealth. Save at least 10 percent of what you earn each week, and put it into a separate account. When you are ready to celebrate you, this money will be there ready to use. This habit will help you develop a new, healthy mind-set. This is your third affirmation to remind yourself of every day. Keep writing the affirmations in your journal. _____
_____
_____
_____
_____

_____The movement of the week will stimulate the elimination organs. This week's movement is thirty minutes of exercise for five days. Continue stretching for ten minutes before and after you exercise. Turn on the music, get up, and dance! Make an appointment for a massage, or get into a sauna this week._____
_____
_____

_____The mindful meditation of the week is a visualization exercise. What do you envision the end result of this program looking like for you? How will the people in your life celebrate you? Do you just want to feel better in your clothes? Be really clear about your goals; visualize every detail. How will you feel? Dig deeper and really examine your feelings. What do you want six months from now to look like for you? How about one year from now?

_____

_____

_____

_____

_____

_____

Daily Checklist—Week Three

_____Food for the week is purchased.
_____Stay focused on the Mindful-Eating Program.
_____Kitchen is organized for the week.

Wake up
_____Drink a cup of warm water with fresh lemon squeezed into it.
_____Do your mindful meditation of the week.

Breakfast
_____Probiotics supplements
_____Omega-3 fatty acid (either two to three tablespoons of ground flaxseed or fish oil)
_____Fiber
_____Breakfast choice from week three options_____

_____

_____Drink eight ounces of water or herbal tea.
_____Use coconut milk or almond milk instead of cow's milk.
_____Record your drink and food intake in your handbook._____

_____

Snack

_____Drink more water; try to drink sixteen ounces more before lunch.

_____Eat from the approved snack list. _____

Lunch

_____Lunch choice from week three options_____

_____

_____Drink eight ounces more of water.

_____Get outside for at least ten minutes to get some fresh air, or take a walk to visit with someone on a different floor of your office.

_____Record your drink and food intake in your handbook. _____

_____

Midafternoon Snack

_____Eat from the approved snack list. _____

_____Drink sixteen ounces of water, or more, before dinner.

Dinner

_____Dinner choices from week three options _____

_____

_____Drink eight ounces of water after dinner

Bedtime

_____The mindful meditation of the week is a visualization exercise. What do you envision the end result of this program looking like for you? How will the people in your life celebrate you? Do you just want to feel better in your clothes? Be really clear about your goals; visualize every detail. How will you feel? Dig deeper and really examine your feelings. What do you want six months from now to look like for you? How about one year from now?_____

_____

_____

_____

_____

_____

_____The journal exercise of the week is to write down your visu-
alization exercise. Remember to be very specific. At the week's end,
journal about your greatest accomplishment of the week, the biggest
challenge you had this week, and what your main health concern is at
this time. _____

_____
_____
_____
_____
_____
_____
_____
_____
_____
_____
_____
_____
_____
_____
_____
_____
_____
_____
_____
_____
_____
_____
_____
_____
_____
_____
_____

Week Three—Day Three

Revisit your personal, positive goals. _____
_____
_____
_____

Revisit your professional, positive goals. _____
_____
_____
_____

_____Your positive affirmation of the week concerns your career or occupation The principle you will be putting into practice is "*a part of all I earn is mine to keep*". This principle is based on paying yourself first as you work toward accumulating wealth. Save at least 10 percent of what you earn each week, and put it into a separate account. When you are ready to celebrate you, this money will be there ready to use. This habit will help you develop a new, healthy mind-set. This is your third affirmation to remind yourself of every day. Keep writing the affirmations in your journal. _____
_____
_____
_____

_____The movement of the week will stimulate the elimination organs. This week's movement is thirty minutes of exercise for five days. Continue stretching for ten minutes before and after you exercise. Turn on the music, get up, and dance! Make an appointment for a massage, or get into a sauna this week._____
_____
_____

_____The mindful meditation of the week is a visualization exercise. What do you envision the end result of this program looking like for you? How will the people in your life celebrate you? Do you just want to feel better in your clothes? Be really clear about your goals; visualize every detail. How will you feel? Dig deeper and really examine your feelings. What do you want six months from now to look like for you? How about one year from now? _____

_____

_____

_____

_____

_____

_____

Daily Checklist—Week Three

_____Food for the week is purchased.

_____Stay focused on the Mindful-Eating Program.

_____Kitchen is organized for the week.

Wake up

_____Drink a cup of warm water with fresh lemon squeezed into it.

_____Do your mindful meditation of the week.

Breakfast

_____Probiotics supplements

_____Omega-3 fatty acid (either two to three tablespoons of ground flaxseed or fish oil)

_____Fiber

_____Breakfast choice from week three options_____

_____

_____Drink eight ounces of water or herbal tea.

_____Use coconut milk or almond milk instead of cow's milk.

_____Record your drink and food intake in your handbook. _____

_____

_____

Snack

_____Drink more water; try to drink sixteen ounces more before lunch.

_____Eat from the approved snack list.

Lunch

_____Lunch choice from week three options_____

_____

_____Drink eight ounces more of water.

_____Get outside for at least ten minutes to get some fresh air, or take a walk to visit with someone on a different floor of your office.

_____Record your drink and food intake in your handbook. _____

_____

Midafternoon Snack

_____Eat from the approved snack list. _____

_____Drink sixteen ounces of water, or more, before dinner.

Dinner

_____Dinner choices from week three options _____

_____

_____Drink eight ounces of water after dinner

Bedtime

_____ The mindful meditation of the week is a visualization exercise. What do you envision the end result of this program looking like for you? How will the people in your life celebrate you? Do you just want to feel better in your clothes? Be really clear about your goals; visualize every detail. How will you feel? Dig deeper and really examine your feelings. What do you want six months from now to look like for you? How about one year from now?_____

_____

_____

_____

_____

_____The journal exercise of the week is to write down your visualization exercise. Remember to be very specific. At the week's end, journal about your greatest accomplishment of the week, the biggest challenge you had this week, and what your main health concern is at this time. _____

_____

_____

_____

_____

_____

_____

_____

_____

_____

_____

_____

_____

_____

_____

_____

_____

_____

_____

_____

_____

_____

_____

_____

_____

_____

_____

_____

_____

Week Three—Day Four

Revisit your personal, positive goals. _____
_____
_____
_____

Revisit your professional, positive goals. _____
_____
_____
_____

_____Your positive affirmation of the week concerns your career or occupation The principle you will be putting into practice is "*a part of all I earn is mine to keep*". This principle is based on paying yourself first as you work toward accumulating wealth. Save at least 10 percent of what you earn each week, and put it into a separate account. When you are ready to celebrate you, this money will be there ready to use. This habit will help you develop a new, healthy mind-set. This is your third affirmation to remind yourself of every day. Keep writing the affirmations in your journal._____
_____
_____
_____

_____The movement of the week will stimulate the elimination organs. This week's movement is thirty minutes of exercise for five days. Continue stretching for ten minutes before and after you exercise. Turn on the music, get up, and dance! Make an appointment for a massage, or get into a sauna this week._____
_____
_____

_____The mindful meditation of the week is a visualization exercise. What do you envision the end result of this program looking like for you? How will the people in your life celebrate you? Do you just want to feel better in your clothes? Be really clear about your goals; visualize every detail. How will you feel? Dig deeper and really examine your feelings. What do you want six months from now to look like for you? How about one year from now?

_____

_____

_____

_____

_____

_____

_____

Daily Checklist—Week Three

_____Food for the week is purchased.
_____Stay focused on the Mindful-Eating Program.
_____Kitchen is organized for the week.

Wake up
_____Drink a cup of warm water with fresh lemon squeezed into it.
_____Do your mindful meditation of the week.

Breakfast
_____Probiotics supplements
_____Omega-3 fatty acid (either two to three tablespoons of ground flaxseed or fish oil)
_____Fiber
_____Breakfast choice from week three options_____

_____

_____Drink eight ounces of water or herbal tea.
_____Use coconut milk or almond milk instead of cow's milk.

_____Record your drink and food intake in your handbook. _____

Snack
_____Drink more water; try to drink sixteen ounces more before lunch.
_____Eat from the approved snack list.

Lunch
_____Lunch choice from week three options_____

_____Drink eight ounces more of water.
_____Get outside for at least ten minutes to get some fresh air, or take a walk to visit with someone on a different floor of your office.
_____Record your drink and food intake in your handbook. _____

Midafternoon Snack
_____Eat from the approved snack list. _____
_____Drink sixteen ounces of water, or more, before dinner.

Dinner
_____Dinner choices from week three options _____

_____Drink eight ounces of water after dinner

Bedtime
_____ The mindful meditation of the week is a visualization exercise. What do you envision the end result of this program looking like for you? How will the people in your life celebrate you? Do you just want to feel better in your clothes? Be really clear about your goals; visualize every detail. How will you feel? Dig deeper and really examine your feelings. What do you want six months from now to look like for you? How about one year from now?_____

_____

_____

_____

_____

_____The journal exercise of the week is to write down your visualization exercise. Remember to be very specific. At the week's end, journal about your greatest accomplishment of the week, the biggest challenge you had this week, and what your main health concern is at this time. _____

_____

_____

_____

_____

_____

_____

_____

_____

_____

_____

_____

_____

_____

_____

_____

_____

_____

_____

_____

_____

_____

Week Three—Day Five

Revisit your personal, positive goals. _____

_____

_____

_____

_____

Revisit your professional, positive goals. _____

_____

_____

_____

_____

_____Your positive affirmation of the week concerns your career or occupation The principle you will be putting into practice is "*a part of all I earn is mine to keep.*" This principle is based on paying yourself first as you work toward accumulating wealth. Save at least 10 percent of what you earn each week, and put it into a separate account. When you are ready to celebrate you, this money will be there ready to use. This habit will help you develop a new, healthy mind-set. This is your third affirmation to remind yourself of every day. Keep writing the affirmations in your journal. _____

_____

_____

_____

_____

_____

_____The movement of the week will stimulate the elimination organs. This week's movement is thirty minutes of exercise for five days. Continue stretching for ten minutes before and after you exercise. Turn on the music, get up, and dance! Make an appointment for a massage, or get into a sauna this week._____

_____

_____

_____The mindful meditation of the week is a visualization exercise. What do you envision the end result of this program looking like for you? How will the people in your life celebrate you? Do you just want to feel better in your clothes? Be really clear about your goals; visualize every detail. How will you feel? Dig deeper and really examine your feelings. What do you want six months from now to look like for you? How about one year from now? _____

_____

_____

_____

_____

_____

_____

_____

_____

Daily Checklist—Week Three

_____Food for the week is purchased.
_____Stay focused on the Mindful-Eating Program.
_____Kitchen is organized for the week.

Wake up
_____Drink a cup of warm water with fresh lemon squeezed into it.
_____Do your mindful meditation of the week.

Breakfast
_____Probiotics supplements
_____Omega-3 fatty acid (either two to three tablespoons of ground flaxseed or fish oil)
_____Fiber

_____Breakfast choice from week three options_____

_____Drink eight ounces of water or herbal tea.

_____Use coconut milk or almond milk instead of cow's milk.

_____Record your drink and food intake in your handbook. _____

Snack

_____Drink more water; try to drink sixteen ounces more before lunch.

_____Eat from the approved snack list. _____

Lunch

_____Lunch choice from week three options_____

_____Drink eight ounces more of water.

_____Get outside for at least ten minutes to get some fresh air, or take a walk to visit with someone on a different floor of your office.

_____Record your drink and food intake in your handbook. _____

Midafternoon Snack

_____Eat from the approved snack list._____

_____Drink sixteen ounces of water, or more, before dinner.

Dinner

_____Dinner choices from week three options _____

_____Drink eight ounces of water after dinner

Bedtime

_____ The mindful meditation of the week is a visualization exercise. What do you envision the end result of this program looking like for you? How will the people in your life celebrate you? Do you just want to feel better in your clothes? Be really clear about your goals; visualize every detail. How will you feel? Dig deeper and really examine your feelings. What do you want six months from now to look like for you? How about one year from now?_____

_____

_____

_____

_____

_____

_____

_____

_____

_____

_____

_____The journal exercise of the week is to write down your visualization exercise. Remember to be very specific. At the week's end, journal about your greatest accomplishment of the week, the biggest challenge you had this week, and what your main health concern is at this time. _____

_____

_____

_____

_____

_____

_____

_____

_____

_____

_____

_____

_____

_____

Week Three—Day Six

Revisit your personal, positive goals. _____

_____

_____

_____

Revisit your professional, positive goals. _____

_____

_____

_____

_____Your positive affirmation of the week concerns your career or occupation The principle you will be putting into practice is "*a part of all I earn is mine to keep*". This principle is based on paying yourself first as you work toward accumulating wealth. Save at least 10 percent of what you earn each week, and put it into a separate account. When you are ready to celebrate you, this money will be there ready to use. This habit will help you develop a new, healthy mind-set. This is your third affirmation to remind yourself of every day. Keep writing the affirmations in your journal. _____

_____

_____

_____

_____

_____The movement of the week will stimulate the elimination organs. This week's movement is thirty minutes of exercise for five days. Continue stretching for ten minutes before and after you exercise. Turn on the music, get up, and dance! Make an appointment for a massage, or get into a sauna this week._____

_____

_____

_____

_____The mindful meditation of the week is a visualization exercise. What do you envision the end result of this program looking like for you? How will the people in your life celebrate you? Do you just want to feel better in your clothes? Be really clear about your goals; visualize every detail. How will you feel? Dig deeper and really examine your feelings. What do you want six months from now to look like for you? How about one year from now?

_____

_____

_____

_____

_____

_____

Daily Checklist—Week Three

_____Food for the week is purchased.
_____Stay focused on the Mindful-Eating Program.
_____Kitchen is organized for the week.

Wake up
_____Drink a cup of warm water with fresh lemon squeezed into it.
_____Do your mindful meditation of the week.

Breakfast
_____Probiotics supplements
_____Omega-3 fatty acid (either two to three tablespoons of ground flaxseed or fish oil)
_____Fiber
_____Breakfast choice from week three options_____

_____

_____Drink eight ounces of water or herbal tea.
_____Use coconut milk or almond milk instead of cow's milk.
_____Record your drink and food intake in your handbook. _____

_____

Snack

_____Drink more water; try to drink sixteen ounces more before lunch.

_____Eat from the approved snack list.

Lunch

_____Lunch choice from week three options_____

_____

_____Drink eight ounces more of water.

_____Get outside for at least ten minutes to get some fresh air, or take a walk to visit with someone on a different floor of your office.

_____Record your drink and food intake in your handbook. _____

_____

Midafternoon Snack

_____Eat from the approved snack list. _____

_____Drink sixteen ounces of water, or more, before dinner.

Dinner

_____Dinner choices from week three options _____

_____

_____Drink eight ounces of water after dinner

Bedtime

_____ The mindful meditation of the week is a visualization exercise. What do you envision the end result of this program looking like for you? How will the people in your life celebrate you? Do you just want to feel better in your clothes? Be really clear about your goals; visualize every detail. How will you feel? Dig deeper and really examine your feelings. What do you want six months from now to look like for you? How about one year from now?_____

_____
_____
_____
_____
_____

_____

_____

_____

_____

_____

_____

_____The journal exercise of the week is to write down your visualization exercise. Remember to be very specific. At the week's end, journal about your greatest accomplishment of the week, the biggest challenge you had this week, and what your main health concern is at this time. _____

_____

_____

_____

_____

_____

_____

_____

_____

_____

_____

_____

_____

_____

_____

_____

_____

_____

_____

_____

Week Three—Day Seven

Revisit your personal, positive goals._____
_____
_____
_____

Revisit your professional, positive goals. _____
_____
_____
_____

_____Your positive affirmation of the week concerns your career or occupation The principle you will be putting into practice is *"a part of all I earn is mine to keep"*. This principle is based on paying yourself first as you work toward accumulating wealth. Save at least 10 percent of what you earn each week, and put it into a separate account. When you are ready to celebrate you, this money will be there ready to use. This habit will help you develop a new, healthy mind-set. This is your third affirmation to remind yourself of every day. Keep writing the affirmations in your journal. _____
_____
_____
_____
_____

_____The movement of the week will stimulate the elimination organs. This week's movement is thirty minutes of exercise for five days. Continue stretching for ten minutes before and after you exercise. Turn on the music, get up, and dance! Make an appointment for a massage, or get into a sauna this week._____
_____
_____

_____The mindful meditation of the week is a visualization exercise. What do you envision the end result of this program looking like for you? How will the people in your life celebrate you? Do you just want to feel better in your clothes? Be really clear about your goals; visualize every detail. How will you feel? Dig deeper and really examine your feelings. What do you want six months from now to look like for you? How about one year from now?

_____

_____

_____

_____

_____

_____

Daily Checklist—Week Three

_____Food for the week is purchased.

_____Stay focused on the Mindful-Eating Program.

_____Kitchen is organized for the week.

Wake up

_____Drink a cup of warm water with fresh lemon squeezed into it.

_____Do your mindful meditation of the week.

Breakfast

_____Probiotics supplements

_____Omega-3 fatty acid (either two to three tablespoons of ground flaxseed or fish oil)

_____Fiber

_____Breakfast choice from week three options_____

_____

_____Drink eight ounces of water or herbal tea.

_____Use coconut milk or almond milk instead of cow's milk.

_____Record your drink and food intake in your handbook._____

Snack

_____Drink more water; try to drink sixteen ounces more before lunch.

_____Eat from the approved snack list._____

Lunch

_____Lunch choice from week three options_____

_____

_____Drink eight ounces more of water.

_____Get outside for at least ten minutes to get some fresh air, or take a walk to visit with someone on a different floor of your office.

_____Record your drink and food intake in your handbook. _____

_____

Midafternoon Snack

_____Eat from the approved snack list. _____

_____Drink sixteen ounces of water, or more, before dinner.

Dinner

_____Dinner choices from week three options _____

_____

_____Drink eight ounces of water after dinner

Bedtime

_____The mindful meditation of the week is a visualization exercise. What do you envision the end result of this program looking like for you? How will the people in your life celebrate you? Do you just want to feel better in your clothes? Be really clear about your goals; visualize every detail. How will you feel? Dig deeper and really examine your feelings. What do you want six months from now to look like for you? How about one year from now?_____

_____

_____

_____

_____

_____The journal exercise of the week is to write down your visualization exercise. Remember to be very specific. At the week's end, journal about your greatest accomplishment of the week, the biggest challenge you had this week, and what your main health concern is at this time. _____

_____

_____

_____

_____

_____

_____

_____

_____

_____

_____

_____

_____

_____

_____

_____

_____

_____

_____

_____

_____

_____

Current weight?_____

Measurements of waist?_____ Hips?_____ Thigh?_____

SHOPPING LIST— WEEK FOUR

<u>Fruits and Vegetables</u>
Yellow bell pepper
Red bell pepper
Zucchini
Celery
Scallions
Lime
Red onion
White onion
Jalapeno
Baby spinach
Arugula
Carrots
Yukon Gold potatoes
Kale
Golden beets
Cauliflower

<u>Nuts, Seeds, and Fresh Herbs</u>
(unsalted nuts, raw, dry roasted, or nut butter)
Slivered almonds

Fresh basil
Fresh thyme
Fresh cilantro
Cumin
Garlic cloves

Protein
(organic, free range, or wild)
Tinned sardines, broken into pieces

Beans
Black beans, cooked and drained
Canned navy beans
Frozen, shelled edamame

Pantry
Quinoa
Whole-wheat spaghetti

Condiments
Extra-virgin olive oil
Red-wine vinegar

Spices
Red-pepper flakes

Week Four—Day One

This is a big week; you are one week away from completing the Mindful-Eating Program. Revisit the health questionnaire you filled out at the beginning of the program. Over the past three weeks, you've probably found you have lost some of those symptoms and also lost some weight. You also may have gained better sleep and increased energy and may have started thinking more clearly. Finish strong this last week, with no processed foods or drinks. If you normally eat animal proteins, it's OK to add those back on your plate, but do opt for organic/sustainable options when possible.

Let's talk about reintroducing foods to your clean, healthy, energized body. Don't go crazy by reintroducing too many of the foods all at once that you have been avoiding for the past three weeks. Go slowly, and reintroduce foods one by one; you will be able to see how your body responds. This can be a helpful way to find out if you are sensitive to foods that commonly cause inflammation and fatigue. If you find a food that definitely seems to cause symptoms, exclude it from your plate for two to three months, and then eat it again. Symptoms can be bloating, nausea, constipation, increased heart rate, unpleasant mood changes, depression, poor concentration, headaches, fluid retention, lethargy, and joint aches or pains. If you have a reaction, then immediately stop eating that food. Record all of your symptoms and your body's reactions to these foods. If you have a reaction, drink lots of water to flush out your system. If you experience no reaction, then move on with lunch and dinner.

Revisit your personal, positive goals. _____

_____

_____

_____

Revisit your professional, positive goals. _____

_____

_____

_____

_____Your positive affirmation of the week concerns your spiritual beliefs or practices. Say, "Thank you, ____, for blessing me with abundance every day in every way." This affirmation is very powerful, and you can actually give this one some rhythm. _____

_____

_____

_____

_____The movement of the week is thirty minutes of exercise for five days; keep stretching for ten minutes before and after exercise. Turn on the music, get up, and dance! Have a massage and a sauna this week. Consider starting yoga. Yoga is an amazing way to exercise. It's a gentle exercise that can aid in eliminating waste, and it's great for stress and weight loss. In order to experience the benefits of yoga fully, you will need to attend a class. _____

_____

_____

_____

Mindful Daily Checklist—Week Four

_____Follow the Mindful-Eating Program completely.
_____Exercise daily (walk, run, swim, yoga, Pilates, tai-chi, bike, dance, walk steps).
_____Food for the week is purchased.
_____Kitchen is organized for the week.

Wake up
_____Drink a cup of warm water with fresh lemon squeezed into it.
_____Do the mindful meditation of the week.

Breakfast

_____Probiotics supplements

_____Omega-3 fatty acid (either two to three tablespoons of ground flaxseed or fish oil)

_____Fiber

_____Breakfast choice from week four or week three options_____

_____

_____Drink eight ounces of water or herbal tea.

_____Use coconut milk or almond milk instead of cow's milk.

_____Record your drink and food intake in your handbook. _____

_____

Snack

_____Drink more water; try to drink sixteen ounces more before lunch.

_____Eat from the approved snack list._____

Lunch

_____Lunch choice from week four options. _____

_____

_____Drink eight ounces more of water.

_____Get outside for at least ten minutes to get some fresh air, or take a walk to visit with someone on a different floor.

_____Record your drink and food intake in your handbook. _____

_____

Midafternoon Snack

_____Eat from the approved snack list. _____

_____Drink sixteen ounces more of water before dinner.

Dinner

_____Dinner choices from week four options. _____

_____

_____Drink eight ounces of water after dinner.

Bedtime

_____Complete the mindful meditation of the week. Your mindful meditation assignment this week is to sit for fifteen minutes with your eyes closed, and be fully present with your new healthy body by acknowledging your heart beating, your lungs breathing, and the sounds around you. _____

_____

_____

_____

_____The journal exercise of the week is to take a moment to check in with yourself. What are your intentions or goals for the upcoming days, weeks, and months of the year? What is good in your life right now, and what would you like to see change? Create two to five action steps to help you achieve these goals or intentions. You will feel more centered and less stressed and have more energy to create balance and enjoy your new healthy lifestyle. _____

_____

_____

_____

_____

_____

_____

_____

_____

_____

_____

_____

_____

_____

_____

_____

_____

Week Four—Day Two

This is a big week; you are one week away from completing the Mindful-Eating Program. Revisit the health questionnaire you filled out at the beginning of the program. Over the past three weeks, you've probably found you have lost some of those symptoms and also lost some weight. You also may have gained better sleep and increased energy and may have started thinking more clearly. Finish strong this last week, with no processed foods or drinks. If you normally eat animal proteins, it's OK to add those back on your plate, but do opt for organic/sustainable options when possible.

Revisit your personal, positive goals. _____

_____

_____

_____

Revisit your professional, positive goals. _____

_____

_____

_____

_____Your positive affirmation of the week concerns your spiritual beliefs or practices. Say, "Thank you, ____, for blessing me with abundance every day in every way." This affirmation is very powerful, and you can actually give this one some rhythm. _____

_____

_____

_____

_____

_____The movement of the week is thirty minutes of exercise for five days; keep stretching for ten minutes before and after you exercise. Turn on the music, get up, and dance! Have a massage and a sauna this week. Consider starting yoga. Yoga is an amazing way to exercise.

It's a gentle exercise that can aid in eliminating waste, and it's great for stress and weight loss. In order to experience the benefits of yoga fully, you will need to attend a class. _____

_____

_____

_____

Mindful Daily Checklist—Week Four

_____Follow the Mindful-Eating Program completely.

_____Exercise daily (walk, run, swim, yoga, Pilates, tai-chi, bike, dance, walk steps).

_____Food for the week is purchased.

_____Kitchen is organized for the week.

Wake up

_____Drink a cup of warm water with fresh lemon squeezed into it.

_____Do the mindful meditation of the week.

Breakfast

_____Probiotics supplements

_____Omega-3 fatty acid (either two to three tablespoons of ground flaxseed or fish oil)

_____Fiber

_____Breakfast choice from week four or week three options. _____

_____

_____Drink eight ounces of water or herbal tea.

_____Use coconut milk or almond milk instead of cow's milk.

_____Record your drink and food intake in your handbook. _____

_____

Snack

_____Drink more water; try to drink sixteen ounces more before lunch.

_____Eat from the approved snack list. _____

Lunch

_____Lunch choice from week four options_____

_____

_____Drink eight ounces more of water.

_____Get outside for at least ten minutes to get some fresh air, or take a walk to visit with someone on a different floor.

_____Record your drink and food intake in your handbook. _____

_____

Midafternoon Snack

_____Eat from the approved snack list. _____

_____Drink sixteen ounces more of water before dinner.

Dinner

_____Dinner choices from week four options. _____

_____

_____Drink eight ounces of water after dinner.

Bedtime

_____Complete the mindful meditation of the week. Your mindful meditation assignment this week is to sit for fifteen minutes with your eyes closed, and be fully present with your new healthy body by acknowledging your heart beating, your lungs breathing, and the sounds around you. _____

_____

_____

_____

_____

_____The journal exercise of the week is to take a moment to check in with yourself. What are your intentions or goals for the upcoming days, weeks, and months of the year? What is good in your life right now, and what would you like to see change? Create two to five action steps to help you achieve these goals or intentions. You will feel more

centered and less stressed and have more energy to create balance and enjoy your new healthy lifestyle. _____

_____

_____

_____

_____

_____

_____

_____

_____

_____

_____

_____

_____

_____

_____

_____

_____

_____

_____

_____

_____

_____

_____

_____

_____

_____

_____

_____

_____

_____

_____

_____

_____

_____

Week Four—Day Three

This is a big week; you are one week away from completing the Mindful-Eating Program. Revisit the health questionnaire you filled out at the beginning of the program. Over the past three weeks, you've probably found you have lost some of those symptoms and also lost some weight. You also may have gained better sleep and increased energy and may have started thinking more clearly. Finish strong this last week, with no processed foods or drinks. If you normally eat animal proteins, it's OK to add those back on your plate, but do opt for organic/sustainable options when possible.

Revisit your personal, positive goals. _____

_____

_____

_____

Revisit your professional, positive goals. _____

_____

_____

_____

_____Your positive affirmation of the week concerns your spiritual beliefs or practices. Say, "Thank you, _____, for blessing me with abundance every day in every way." This affirmation is very powerful, and you can actually give this one some rhythm. _____

_____

_____

_____

_____

_____The movement of the week is thirty minutes of exercise for five days; keep stretching for ten minutes before and after you exercise. Turn on the music, get up, and dance! Have a massage and a sauna this week. Consider starting yoga. Yoga is an amazing way to exercise.

It's a gentle exercise that can aid in eliminating waste, and it's great for stress and weight loss. In order to experience the benefits of yoga fully, you will need to attend a class. _____

_____

_____

_____

Mindful Daily Checklist—Week Four

_____Follow the Mindful-Eating Program completely.

_____Exercise daily (walk, run, swim, yoga, Pilates, tai-chi, bike, dance, walk steps).

_____Food for the week is purchased.

_____Kitchen is organized for the week.

Wake up

_____Drink a cup of warm water with fresh lemon squeezed into it.

_____Do the mindful meditation of the week.

Breakfast

_____Probiotics supplements

_____Omega-3 fatty acid (either two to three tablespoons of ground flaxseed or fish oil)

_____Fiber

_____Breakfast choice from week four or week three options _____

_____

_____Drink eight ounces of water or herbal tea.

_____Use coconut milk or almond milk instead of cow's milk.

_____Record your drink and food intact in your handbook. _____

_____

Snack

_____Drink more water; try to drink sixteen ounces more before lunch.

_____Eat from the approved snack list. _____

Lunch

_____Lunch choice from week four options _____

_____

_____Drink eight ounces more of water.

_____Get outside for at least ten minutes to get some fresh air, or take a walk to visit with someone on a different floor.

_____Record your drink and food intact in your handbook. _____

_____

Midafternoon Snack

_____Eat from the approved snack list. _____

_____Drink sixteen ounces more of water before dinner.

Dinner

_____Dinner choices from week four options. _____

_____

_____Drink eight ounces of water after dinner.

Bedtime

_____Complete the mindful meditation of the week. Your mindful meditation assignment this week is to sit for fifteen minutes with your eyes closed, and be fully present with your new healthy body by acknowledging your heart beating, your lungs breathing, and the sounds around you. _____

_____

_____

_____

_____The journal exercise of the week is to take a moment to check in with yourself. What are your intentions or goals for the upcoming days, weeks, and months of the year? What is good in your life right now, and what would you like to see change? Create two to five action steps to help you achieve these goals or intentions. You will feel more

centered and less stressed and have more energy to create balance and enjoy your new healthy lifestyle._____

_____
_____
_____
_____
_____
_____
_____
_____
_____
_____
_____
_____
_____
_____
_____
_____
_____
_____
_____
_____
_____
_____
_____
_____
_____
_____
_____
_____
_____
_____
_____
_____
_____
_____
_____
_____

Week Four—Day Four

This is a big week; you are one week away from completing the Mindful-Eating Program. Revisit the health questionnaire you filled out at the beginning of the program. Over the past three weeks, you've probably found you have lost some of those symptoms and also lost some weight. You also may have gained better sleep and increased energy and may have started thinking more clearly. Finish strong this last week, with no processed foods or drinks. If you normally eat animal proteins, it's OK to add those back on your plate, but do opt for organic/sustainable options when possible.

Revisit your personal, positive goals. _____

_____

_____

_____

Revisit your professional, positive goals. _____

_____

_____

_____

_____Your positive affirmation of the week concerns your spiritual beliefs or practices. Say, "Thank you, _____, for blessing me with abundance every day in every way." This affirmation is very powerful, and you can actually give this one some rhythm. _____

_____

_____

_____

_____

_____The movement of the week is thirty minutes of exercise for five days; keep stretching for ten minutes before and after you exercise. Turn on the music, get up, and dance! Have a massage and a sauna this week. Consider starting yoga. Yoga is an amazing way to exercise.

It's a gentle exercise that can aid in eliminating waste, and it's great for stress and weight loss. In order to experience the benefits of yoga fully, you will need to attend a class. _____

_____

_____

_____

Mindful Daily Checklist—Week Four

_____Follow the Mindful-Eating Program completely.

_____Exercise daily (walk, run, swim, yoga, Pilates, tai-chi, bike, dance, walk steps).

_____Food for the week is purchased.

_____Kitchen is organized for the week.

Wake up

_____Drink a cup of warm water with fresh lemon squeezed into it.

_____Do the mindful meditation of the week.

Breakfast

_____Probiotics supplements

_____Omega-3 fatty acid (either two to three tablespoons of ground flaxseed or fish oil)

_____Fiber

_____Breakfast choice from week four or week three options _____

_____

_____Drink eight ounces of water or herbal tea.

_____Use coconut milk or almond milk instead of cow's milk.

_____Record your drink and food intact in your handbook._____

_____

Snack

_____Drink more water; try to drink sixteen ounces more before lunch.

_____Eat from the approved snack list._____

Lunch

_____Lunch choice from week four options_____

_____

_____Drink eight ounces more of water.
_____Get outside for at least ten minutes to get some fresh air, or take a walk to visit with someone on a different floor.
_____Record your drink and food intact in your handbook. _____

_____

Midafternoon Snack
_____Eat from the approved snack list._____
_____Drink sixteen ounces more of water before dinner.

Dinner
_____Dinner choices from week four options. _____

_____

_____Drink eight ounces of water after dinner.

Bedtime
_____Complete the mindful meditation of the week. Your mindful meditation assignment this week is to sit for fifteen minutes with your eyes closed, and be fully present with your new healthy body by acknowledging your heart beating, your lungs breathing, and the sounds around you. _____

_____

_____

_____

_____The journal exercise of the week is to take a moment to check in with yourself. What are your intentions or goals for the upcoming days, weeks, and months of the year? What is good in your life right now, and what would you like to see change? Create two to five action steps to help you achieve these goals or intentions. You will feel more

centered and less stressed and have more energy to create balance and enjoy your new healthy lifestyle._____

_____

_____

_____

_____

_____

_____

_____

_____

_____

_____

_____

_____

_____

_____

_____

_____

_____

_____

_____

_____

_____

_____

_____

_____

_____

_____

_____

_____

_____

_____

_____

_____

_____

Week Four—Day Five

This is a big week; you are one week away from completing the Mindful-Eating Program. Revisit the health questionnaire you filled out at the beginning of the program. Over the past three weeks, you've probably found you have lost some of those symptoms and also lost some weight. You also may have gained better sleep and increased energy and may have started thinking more clearly. Finish strong this last week, with no processed foods or drinks. If you normally eat animal proteins, it's OK to add those back on your plate, but do opt for organic/sustainable options when possible.

Revisit your personal, positive goals. _____
_____
_____
_____

Revisit your professional, positive goals. _____
_____
_____
_____

_____Your positive affirmation of the week concerns your spiritual beliefs or practices. Say, "Thank you, ____, for blessing me with abundance every day in every way." This affirmation is very powerful, and you can actually give this one some rhythm. _____
_____
_____
_____

_____The movement of the week is thirty minutes of exercise for five days; keep stretching for ten minutes before and after you exercise. Turn on the music, get up, and dance! By this time you should be up to five pounds with your hand weights. Have a massage and a sauna this week. Consider starting yoga. Yoga is an amazing way to exercise. It's a gentle exercise that can aid in eliminating waste, and it's great for stress and weight loss. In order to experience the benefits of yoga fully, you will need to attend a class. _____

_____

_____

_____

Mindful Daily Checklist—Week Four

_____Follow the Mindful-Eating Program completely.

_____Exercise daily (walk, run, swim, yoga, Pilates, tai-chi, bike, dance, walk steps).

_____Food for the week is purchased.

_____Kitchen is organized for the week.

Wake up

_____Drink a cup of warm water with fresh lemon squeezed into it.

_____Do the mindful meditation of the week.

Breakfast

_____Probiotics supplements

_____Omega-3 fatty acid (either two to three tablespoons of ground flaxseed or fish oil)

_____Fiber

_____Breakfast choice from week four or week three options _____

_____

_____Drink eight ounces of water or herbal tea.

_____Use coconut milk or almond milk instead of cow's milk.

_____Record your drink and food intact in your handbook. _____

_____

Snack

_____Drink more water; try to drink sixteen ounces more before lunch.

_____Eat from the approved snack list.

Lunch

_____Lunch choice from week four options _____

_____

_____Drink eight ounces more of water.

_____Get outside for at least ten minutes to get some fresh air, or take a walk to visit with someone on a different floor.

_____Record your drink and food intake in your handbook. _____

_____

Midafternoon Snack

_____Eat from the approved snack list.

_____Drink sixteen ounces more of water before dinner.

Dinner

_____Dinner choices from week four options._____

_____

_____Drink eight ounces of water after dinner.

Bedtime

_____Complete the mindful meditation of the week. Your mindful meditation assignment this week is to sit for fifteen minutes with your eyes closed, and be fully present with your new healthy body by acknowledging your heart beating, your lungs breathing, and the sounds around you. _____

_____

_____

_____The journal exercise of the week is to take a moment to check in with yourself. What are your intentions or goals for the upcoming days, weeks, and months of the year? What is good in your life right now, and what would you like to see change? Create two to five action steps to help you achieve these goals or intentions. You will feel more

centered and less stressed and have more energy to create balance and enjoy your new healthy lifestyle._____

_____

_____

_____

_____

_____

_____

_____

_____

_____

_____

_____

_____

_____

_____

_____

_____

_____

_____

_____

_____

_____

_____

_____

_____

_____

_____

_____

_____

_____

_____

_____

_____

Week Four—Day Six

This is a big week; you are one week away from completing the Mindful-Eating Program. Revisit the health questionnaire you filled out at the beginning of the program. Over the past three weeks, you've probably found you have lost some of those symptoms and also lost some weight. You also may have gained better sleep and increased energy and may have started thinking more clearly. Finish strong this last week, with no processed foods or drinks. If you normally eat animal proteins, it's OK to add those back on your plate, but do opt for organic/sustainable options when possible.

Revisit your personal, positive goals _____
_____
_____
_____

Revisit your professional, positive goals _____
_____
_____
_____

_____Your positive affirmation of the week concerns your spiritual beliefs or practices. Say, "Thank you, ____, for blessing me with abundance every day in every way." This affirmation is very powerful, and you can actually give this one some rhythm. _____
_____
_____
_____

_____The movement of the week is thirty minutes of exercise for five days; keep stretching for ten minutes before and after you exercise. Turn on the music, get up, and dance! Have a massage and a sauna this week. Consider starting yoga. Yoga is an amazing way to exercise.

It's a gentle exercise that can aid in eliminating waste, and it's great for stress and weight loss. In order to experience the benefits of yoga fully, you will need to attend a class. _____

_____

_____

_____

Mindful Daily Checklist—Week Four

_____Follow the Mindful-Eating Program completely.

_____Exercise daily (walk, run, swim, yoga, Pilates, tai-chi, bike, dance, walk steps).

_____Food for the week is purchased.

_____Kitchen is organized for the week.

Wake up

_____Drink a cup of warm water with fresh lemon squeezed into it.

_____Do the mindful meditation of the week.

Breakfast

_____Probiotics supplements

_____Omega-3 fatty acid (either two to three tablespoons of ground flaxseed or fish oil)

_____Fiber

_____Breakfast choice from week four or week three options_____

_____

_____Drink eight ounces of water or herbal tea.

_____Use coconut milk or almond milk instead of cow's milk.

_____Record your drink and food intact in your handbook._____

_____

Snack

_____Drink more water; try to drink sixteen ounces more before lunch.

_____Eat from the approved snack list.

Lunch

_____Lunch choice from week four options _____

_____

_____Drink eight ounces more of water.

_____Get outside for at least ten minutes to get some fresh air, or take a walk to visit with someone on a different floor.

_____Record your drink and food intact in your handbook._____

_____

Midafternoon Snack

_____Eat from the approved snack list. _____

_____Drink sixteen ounces more of water before dinner.

Dinner

_____Dinner choices from week four options. _____

_____

_____Drink eight ounces of water after dinner.

Bedtime

_____Complete the mindful meditation of the week. Your mindful meditation assignment this week is to sit for fifteen minutes with your eyes closed, and be fully present with your new healthy body by acknowledging your heart beating, your lungs breathing, and the sounds around you. _____

_____

_____

_____

_____The journal exercise of the week is to take a moment to check in with yourself. What are your intentions or goals for the upcoming days, weeks, and months of the year? What is good in your life right now, and what would you like to see change? Create two to five action steps to help you achieve these goals or intentions. You will feel more

centered and less stressed and have more energy to create balance and enjoy your new healthy lifestyle._____

_____
_____
_____
_____
_____
_____
_____
_____
_____
_____
_____
_____
_____
_____
_____
_____
_____
_____
_____
_____
_____
_____
_____
_____
_____
_____
_____
_____
_____
_____
_____
_____

Week Four—Day Seven

This is a big week; you are one week away from completing the Mindful-Eating Program. Revisit the health questionnaire you filled out at the beginning of the program. Over the past three weeks, you've probably found you have lost some of those symptoms and also lost some weight. You also may have gained better sleep and increased energy and may have started thinking more clearly. Finish strong this last week, with no processed foods or drinks. If you normally eat animal proteins, it's OK to add those back on your plate, but do opt for organic/sustainable options when possible.

Revisit your personal, positive goals. _____

_____

_____

_____

Revisit your professional, positive goals. _____

_____

_____

_____

_____Your positive affirmation of the week concerns your spiritual beliefs or practices. Say, "Thank you, ____, for blessing me with abundance every day in every way." This affirmation is very powerful, and you can actually give this one some rhythm. _____

_____

_____

_____

_____

_____The movement of the week is thirty minutes of exercise for five days; keep stretching for ten minutes before and after you exercise. Turn on the music, get up, and dance! Have a massage and a sauna this week. Consider starting yoga. Yoga is an amazing way to exercise.

It's a gentle exercise that can aid in eliminating waste, and it's great for stress and weight loss. In order to experience the benefits of yoga fully, you will need to attend a class._____

_____

_____

_____

_____

Mindful Daily Checklist—Week Four

_____Follow the Mindful-Eating Program completely.

_____Exercise daily (walk, run, swim, yoga, Pilates, tai-chi, bike, dance, walk steps).

_____Food for the week is purchased.

_____Kitchen is organized for the week.

Wake up

_____Drink a cup of warm water with fresh lemon squeezed into it.

_____Do the mindful meditation of the week.

Breakfast

_____Probiotics supplements

_____Omega-3 fatty acid (either two to three tablespoons of ground flaxseed or fish oil)

_____Fiber

_____Breakfast choice from week four or week three options _____

_____

_____Drink eight ounces of water or herbal tea.

_____Use coconut milk or almond milk instead of cow's milk.

_____Record your drink and food intact in your handbook._____

_____

Snack

_____Drink more water; try to drink sixteen ounces more before lunch.

_____Eat from the approved snack list. _____

Lunch
_____Lunch choice from week four options _____

_____

_____Drink eight ounces more of water.
_____Get outside for at least ten minutes to get some fresh air, or
take a walk to visit with someone on a different floor.
_____Record your drink and food intact in your handbook. _____

_____

Midafternoon Snack
_____Eat from the approved snack list.
_____Drink sixteen ounces more of water before dinner.

Dinner
_____Dinner choices from week four options. _____

_____

_____Drink eight ounces of water after dinner.

Bedtime
_____Complete the mindful meditation of the week. Your mindful
meditation assignment this week is to sit for fifteen minutes with your
eyes closed, and be fully present with your new healthy body by acknowledging your heart beating, your lungs breathing, and the sounds
around you. _____

_____

_____

_____

_____The journal exercise of the week is to take a moment to check
in with yourself. What are your intentions or goals for the upcoming
days, weeks, and months of the year? What is good in your life right
now, and what would you like to see change? Create two to five action
steps to help you achieve these goals or intentions. You will feel more
centered and less stressed and have more energy to create balance and
enjoy your new healthy lifestyle._____

_____

_____

_____

_____

_____

_____

_____

_____

_____

_____

_____

_____

_____

_____

_____

_____

_____

_____

_____

_____

_____

Current weight? _____

Measurements of waist? _____ Hips? _____ Thigh? _____

What is your goal? _____

Has it changed? _____

_____

_____

_____

_____

_____

Shopping List—
Week Five

Fruits and Vegetables
Fresh fruit (no banana)
Raw vegetable salad-(No Avocados)
Lemons, at least a dozen
Garlic
Extra-virgin olive oil
Steamed vegetables
Smoothie made with fresh vegetable juice or water
Raw organic fruit, in season
Freshly grated cabbage
Carrot
Beets
Fresh vegetable salad or steamed vegetables
Cooked and raw vegetables

Nuts and Seeds
(unsalted, raw, dry roasted, nut butter, or oil)
Ground flaxseed
Flaxseed oil

Pantry
100% pure maple syrup
Green drink powder (health food store)

Vegetarian protein, such as pea or brown rice
Soft grains

Spices
Ground ginger
Cayenne pepper

Week Five—Optional Fasting Phase

Day One—Preparation Day _____
The fasting phase can be the most challenging phase, but it can also be the most productive. If you have completed phases one and two, you should be ready for a one-to-three-day fast. I have included a seven-day fast in this handbook, which can be modified for one to three days. Following the fast, you will return to phase two, weeks three and four of the program, when you are finished.

Revisit your personal, positive goals _____
_____
_____
_____
_____

Revisit your professional, positive goals _____
_____
_____
_____
_____

_____Your positive affirmation of the week is to affirm all four of your previous affirmations every day this week. Write them here in your handbook. _____
_____
_____
_____
_____
_____
_____
_____
_____

_____The movement of the week is light-to-gentle exercise. Yoga is an amazing way to exercise. It's is a gentle exercise that can aid in eliminating waste, and it's great for stress and weight loss. Remember that to experience the benefits of yoga fully, you will need to attend a class. _____

_____

_____

_____

Mindful Daily Checklist—Week Five

_____Follow the Mindful-Eating Program completely.

_____Food for the week is purchased.

_____Kitchen is organized for the week.

Wake up

_____Drink eight ounces of water with the juice from half a lemon squeezed in it.

_____Exercise daily (walk, run, swim, yoga, Pilates, tai-chi, bike, dance, walk steps)

_____Complete your mindful meditation of the week.

Breakfast

_____Omega-3 fatty acid (either two to three tablespoons of ground flaxseed or fish oil)

_____Breakfast choice of fresh, raw fruit (no bananas) or soft, non-gluten grains. _____

_____

_____Drink eight ounces of lemonade that is made according to the recipe in this book.

_____Record your drink and food intake in your handbook_____

_____

Snack

_____Smoothie made with fresh vegetable juice or water, one tablespoon flaxseed meal, one tablespoon flaxseed oil, and greens powder.

_____Drink sixteen ounces more lemonade.

Lunch
_____Raw vegetable salad with lemon dressing
_____Drink twelve ounces lemonade.
_____Get outside for at least ten minutes to get some fresh air, or take a walk to visit with someone on a different floor.
_____Record your drink and food intake in your handbook._____

_____

Midafternoon Snack
_____Smoothie made with fresh vegetable juice or water, one tablespoon flaxseed meal, one tablespoon flaxseed oil, and greens powder.
_____Drink sixteen ounces lemonade before dinner.
Dinner:
_____Dinner plate of steamed vegetables with lemon dressing
_____Drink eight ounces of lemonade

Bedtime
_____The mindful meditation of the week is to sit for fifteen minutes with your eyes closed. Be fully present with your new, healthy body by acknowledging your heart beating, your lungs breathing, and the sounds around you. _____

_____

_____

_____Your journal exercise for the week is to take a moment and check in with yourself. What is good in your life right now, and what would you like to see change? Look over the actions steps from last week; see where you are in regard to taking steps to meet your goals or intentions. _____

_____

_____

_____

_____

Week Five—Day Two

Preparation Day _____

The fasting phase can be the most challenging phase, but it can also be the most productive. If you have completed phases one and two, you should be ready for a one-to-three-day fast. I have included a seven-day fast in this handbook, which can be modified for one to three days. Following the seven-day fast, you will return to phase two, weeks three and four of the program, when you are finished.

Revisit your personal, positive goals._____
_____
_____
_____

Revisit your professional, positive goals._____
_____
_____
_____

_____Your positive affirmation of the week is to affirm all four of your previous affirmations every day this week. Write them here in your handbook. _____
_____
_____
_____
_____
_____
_____
_____
_____
_____

_____The movement of the week is light-to-gentle exercise. Yoga is an amazing way to exercise. It's is a gentle exercise that can aid in eliminating waste, and it's great for stress and weight loss. Remember that to experience the benefits of yoga fully, you will need to attend a class. _____

_____

_____

_____

_____

Mindful Daily Checklist—Week Five
_____Follow the Mindful-Eating Program completely.
_____Food for the week is purchased.
_____Kitchen is organized for the week.

Wake up
_____Drink eight ounces of water with the juice from half a lemon squeezed in it.
_____Exercise daily (walk, run, swim, yoga, Pilates, tai-chi, bike, dance, walk steps).
_____Complete your mindful meditation of the week.

Breakfast
_____Omega-3 fatty acid (either two to three tablespoons of ground flaxseed or fish oil)
_____Breakfast choice of fresh, raw fruit (no bananas) or soft, non-gluten grains. _____

_____

_____Drink eight ounces of lemonade that is made according to the recipe in this book.
_____Record your drink and food intake in your handbook. _____

_____

_____

_____

Snack

_____Smoothie made with fresh vegetable juice or water, one table-spoon flaxseed meal, one tablespoon flaxseed oil, and greens powder.

_____Drink sixteen ounces more lemonade.

Lunch

_____Raw vegetable salad with lemon dressing

_____Drink eight ounces lemonade.

_____Get outside for at least ten minutes to get some fresh air, or take a walk to visit with someone on a different floor, at work.

_____Record your drink and food intake in your handbook. _____

Midafternoon Snack

_____Smoothie made with fresh vegetable juice or water, one table-spoon flaxseed meal, one tablespoon flaxseed oil, and greens powder.

_____Drink sixteen ounces lemonade before dinner.

Dinner:

_____Dinner plate of steamed vegetables with lemon dressing.

_____Drink eight ounces of lemonade

Bedtime

_____The mindful meditation of the week is to sit for fifteen minutes with your eyes closed. Be fully present with your new, healthy body by acknowledging your heart beating, your lungs breathing, and the sounds around you. _____

_____

_____

_____

_____Your journal exercise for the week is to take a moment and check in with yourself. What is good in your life right now, and what would you like to see change? Look over the actions steps from last week; see where you are in regard to taking steps to meet your goals or intentions. _____

Week Five—Day Three

Fasting Day _____

The fasting phase can be the most challenging phase, but it can also be the most productive. If you have completed phases one and two, you should be ready for a one-to-three-day fast. I have included a seven-day fast in this handbook, which can be modified for one to three days. Following the fast, you will return to phase two, weeks three and four of the program, when you are finished.

Revisit your personal, positive goals._____
_____
_____
_____

Revisit your professional, positive goals._____
_____
_____
_____
_____

_____Your positive affirmation of the week is to affirm all four of your previous affirmations every day this week. Write them here in your handbook. _____
_____
_____
_____
_____
_____
_____
_____

_____The movement of the week is light-to-gentle exercise. Yoga is an amazing way to exercise. It's is a gentle exercise that can aid in eliminating waste, and it's great for stress and weight loss. Remember that to experience the benefits of yoga fully, you will need to attend a class. _____

_____

_____

_____

_____

Mindful Daily Checklist for Week Five

_____Follow the Mindful-Eating Program completely.

_____Food for the week is purchased.

_____Kitchen is organized for the week.

Wake up

_____Drink eight ounces of warm water with fresh lemon juice squeezed into it.

_____Complete your mindful meditation of the week.

Breakfast

_____Omega-3 fatty acid (either two to three tablespoons ground flaxseed or fish oil)

_____Drink twelve ounces of lemonade.

_____Daily exercise (walk, run, swim, yoga, Pilates, tai-chi, bike, dance, walk steps)

_____Record your drink intake and your mood in your handbook. __

_____

Lunch

_____Drink twelve ounces of lemonade

_____Get outside for at least ten minutes to get some fresh air, or take a walk to visit with someone on a different floor, at work.

_____Record your drink intake and your mood in your handbook. __

_____

Dinner

_____Drink eight ounces of lemonade.

_____Record your drink intake and your mood in your handbook.___

_____

Bedtime

_____The mindful meditation of the week is to sit for fifteen minutes with your eyes closed. Be fully present with your new, healthy body by acknowledging your heart beating, your lungs breathing, and the sounds around you. _____

_____

_____

_____

_____Your journal exercise for the week is to take a moment and check in with yourself. What is good in your life right now, and what would you like to see change? Look over the actions steps from last week; see where you are in regard to taking steps to meet your goals or intentions. _____

_____

_____

_____

_____

_____

_____

_____

_____

_____

_____

_____

_____

_____

_____

_____

Week Five—Day Four

Fasting Day _____

The fasting phase can be the most challenging phase, but it can also be the most productive. If you have completed phases one and two, you should be ready for a one-to-three-day fast. I have included a seven-day fast in this handbook, which can be modified for one to three days. Following the fast, you will return to phase two, weeks three and four of the program, when you are finished.

Revisit your personal, positive goals. _____
_____
_____
_____

Revisit your professional, positive goals. _____
_____
_____
_____

_____Your positive affirmation of the week is to affirm all four of your previous affirmations every day this week. Write them here in your handbook. _____
_____
_____
_____
_____
_____
_____

_____The movement of the week is light-to-gentle exercise. Yoga is an amazing way to exercise. It's is a gentle exercise that can aid in eliminating waste, and it's great for stress and weight loss. Remember that to experience the benefits of yoga fully, you will need to attend a class. _____

_____

_____

_____

_____

Mindful Daily Checklist for Week Five

_____Follow the Mindful-Eating Program completely.

_____Food for the week is purchased.

_____Kitchen is organized for the week.

Wake up

_____Drink eight ounces of warm water with fresh lemon juice squeezed into it.

_____Complete your mindful meditation of the week.

Breakfast

_____Omega-3 fatty acid (either two to three tablespoons ground flaxseed or fish oil)

_____Drink twelve ounces of lemonade.

_____Daily exercise (walk, run, swim, yoga, Pilates, tai-chi, bike, dance, walk steps)

_____Record your drink intake and your mood in your handbook. __

Lunch

_____Drink twelve ounces of lemonade

_____Get outside for at least ten minutes to get some fresh air, or take a walk to visit with someone on a different floor, at work.

_____Record your drink intake and your mood in your handbook. __

_____

_____

_____

Dinner

_____Drink ten ounces of lemonade.

_____Record your drink intake and your mood in your handbook. __

Bedtime

_____The mindful meditation of the week is to sit for fifteen minutes with your eyes closed. Be fully present with your new, healthy body by acknowledging your heart beating, your lungs breathing, and the sounds around you. _____

_____

_____

_____

_____Your journal exercise for the week is to take a moment and check in with yourself. What is good in your life right now, and what would you like to see change? Look over the actions steps from last week; see where you are in regard to taking steps to meet your goals or intentions. _____

Week Five—Day Five

The fasting phase can be the most challenging phase, but it can also be the most productive. If you have completed phases one and two, you should be ready for a one-to-three-day fast. I have included a seven-day fast in this handbook, which can be modified for one to three days. Following the fast, you will return to phase two, weeks three and four of the program, when you are finished.

Revisit your personal, positive goals. _____
_____
_____
_____

Revisit your professional, positive goals. _____
_____
_____
_____

_____Your positive affirmation of the week is to affirm all four of your previous affirmations every day this week. Write them here in your handbook. _____
_____
_____
_____
_____
_____
_____

_____The movement of the week is light-to-gentle exercise. Yoga is an amazing way to exercise. It's is a gentle exercise that can aid in eliminating waste, and it's great for stress and weight loss. Remember that to experience the benefits of yoga fully, you will need to attend a class. _____
_____

_____

_____

Mindful Daily Checklist for Week Five

_____Follow the Mindful-Eating Program completely.

_____Food for the week is purchased.

_____Kitchen is organized for the week.

Wake up

_____Drink eight ounces of warm water with fresh lemon juice squeezed into it.

_____Complete your mindful meditation of the week.

Breakfast

_____Omega-3 fatty acid (either two to three tablespoons ground flaxseed or fish oil)

_____Drink twelve ounces of lemonade.

_____Daily exercise (walk, run, swim, yoga, Pilates, tai-chi, bike, dance, walk steps)

_____Break the fast with a piece of raw, organic fruit

_____Record your drink and food intake and your mood in your handbook. _____

_____

Lunch

_____Drink twelve ounces of lemonade.

_____Salad with freshly grated cabbage, carrot, and beet tossed with fresh lemon juice

_____Get outside for at least ten minutes to some fresh air, or take a walk to visit with someone on a different floor, at work.

_____Record your drink and food intake and your mood in your handbook. _____

_____

Dinner

_____Drink eight ounces of lemonade.

_____Fresh vegetable salad or steamed vegetables with lemon, garlic, and extra-virgin olive oil dressing

_____Record your drink and food intake and your mood in your handbook. _____

_____

Bedtime

_____The mindful meditation of the week is to sit for fifteen minutes with your eyes closed. Be fully present with your new, healthy body by acknowledging your heart beating, your lungs breathing, and the sounds around you. _____

_____

_____

_____

_____Your journal exercise for the week is to take a moment and check in with yourself. What is good in your life right now, and what would you like to see change? Look over the actions steps from last week; see where you are in regard to taking steps to meet your goals or intentions. _____

_____

_____

_____

_____

_____

_____

_____

_____

_____

_____

_____

Week Five—Day Six

The fasting phase can be the most challenging phase, but it can also be the most productive. If you have completed phases one and two, you should be ready for a one-to-three-day fast. I have included a seven-day fast in this handbook, which can be modified for one to three days. Following the fast, you will return to phase two, weeks three and four of the program, when you are finished.

Revisit your personal, positive goals. _____
_____
_____
_____

Revisit your professional, positive goals. _____
_____
_____
_____

_____Your positive affirmation of the week is to affirm all four of your previous affirmations every day this week. Write them here in your handbook. _____
_____
_____
_____
_____
_____
_____
_____

_____The movement of the week is light-to-gentle exercise. Yoga is an amazing way to exercise. It's is a gentle exercise that can aid in eliminating waste, and it's great for stress and weight loss. Remember that to experience the benefits of yoga fully, you will need to attend

a class. _____
_____
_____
_____

Mindful Daily Checklist for Week Five
_____Follow the Mindful-Eating Program completely.
_____Food for the week is purchased.
_____Kitchen is organized for the week.

Wake up
_____Drink a ten-ounce glass of fresh lemonade.
_____Complete your mindful meditation of the week.

Breakfast
_____Omega-3 fatty acid (either two to three tablespoons ground flaxseed or fish oil)
_____Drink twelve ounces of lemonade.
_____Daily exercise (walk, run, swim, yoga, Pilates, tai-chi, bike, dance, walk steps)
_____Begin adding soft grains, vegetarian protein, and cooked and raw vegetables back into your meals.
_____Piece of fruit, in season
_____Record your drink and food intake and you mood in your handbook. _____
_____

Lunch
_____Drink twelve ounces of lemonade.
_____Begin adding soft grains, vegetarian protein, and cooked and raw vegetables back into your meals.
_____Salad with freshly grated cabbage, carrot, and beet tossed with fresh lemon juice

_____Get outside for at least ten minutes to get some fresh air, or take a walk to visit with someone on a different floor, at work.

_____Record your drink and food intake and your mood in your handbook. _____

_____

Dinner

_____Drink ten ounces of lemonade.

_____Begin adding soft grains, vegetarian protein, and cooked and raw vegetables back into your meals.

_____Fresh vegetable salad or steamed vegetables with lemon, garlic, and extra-virgin olive oil dressing

_____Record your drink and food intake and your mood in your handbook. _____

_____

Bedtime

_____The mindful meditation of the week is to sit for fifteen minutes with your eyes closed. Be fully present with your new, healthy body by acknowledging your heart beating, your lungs breathing, and the sounds around you. _____

_____

_____

_____

_____Your journal exercise for the week is to take a moment and check in with yourself. What is good in your life right now, and what would you like to see change? Look over the actions steps from last week; see where you are in regard to taking steps to meet your goals or intentions. _____

_____

_____

_____

_____

_____

Week Five—Day Seven

The fasting phase can be the most challenging phase, but it can also be the most productive. If you have completed phases one and two, you should be ready for a one-to-three-day fast. I have included a seven-day fast in this handbook, which can be modified for one to three days. Following the fast, you will return to phase two, weeks three and four of the program, when you are finished.

Revisit your personal, positive goals. _____

_____

_____

_____

Revisit your professional, positive goals. _____

_____

_____

_____

_____Your positive affirmation of the week is to affirm all four of your previous affirmations every day this week. Write them here in your handbook. _____

_____

_____

_____

_____

_____

_____

_____

_____

_____The movement of the week is light-to-gentle exercise. Yoga is an amazing way to exercise. It's is a gentle exercise that can aid in eliminating waste, and it's great for stress and weight loss. Remember that to experience the benefits of yoga fully, you will need to attend a class. _____

_____

_____

_____

Mindful Daily Checklist for Week Five

_____Follow the Mindful-Eating Program completely.

_____Food for the week is purchased.

_____Kitchen is organized for the week.

Wake up

_____Drink a ten-ounce glass of fresh lemonade.

_____Complete your mindful meditation of the week.

Breakfast

_____Omega-3 fatty acid (either two to three tablespoons ground flaxseed or fish oil)

_____Drink twelve ounces of lemonade.

_____Daily exercise (walk, run, swim, yoga, Pilates, tai-chi, bike, dance, walk steps)

_____Begin adding soft grains, vegetarian protein, and cooked and raw vegetables back into your meals.

_____Piece of fruit, in season

_____Record your drink and food intake and your mood in your handbook. _____

_____

Lunch

_____Drink twelve ounces of lemonade.

_____Begin adding soft grains, vegetarian protein, and cooked and raw vegetables back into your meals.

_____Salad with freshly grated cabbage, carrot, and beet tossed with fresh lemon juice

_____Get outside for at least ten minutes to get some fresh air, or take a walk to visit with someone on a different floor.

_____Record your drink and food intake and your mood in your handbook.

Dinner

_____Drink eight ounces of lemonade.

_____Continue adding soft grains, vegetarian protein, and cooked and raw vegetables back into your meals.

_____Fresh vegetable salad or steamed vegetables with lemon, garlic, and extra-virgin olive oil dressing

_____Record your drink and food intake and your mood in your handbook. _____

_____

Bedtime

_____The mindful meditation of the week is to sit for fifteen minutes with your eyes closed. Be fully present with your new, healthy body by acknowledging your heart beating, your lungs breathing, and the sounds around you. _____

_____

_____

_____

_____Your journal exercise for the week is to take a moment and check in with yourself. What is good in your life right now, and what would you like to see change? Look over the actions steps from last week; see where you are in regard to taking steps to meet your goals or intentions. _____

_____

_____

_____

_____
_____
_____
_____
_____
_____
_____
_____
_____
_____
_____
_____
_____
_____
_____
_____
_____
_____
_____
_____
_____
_____
_____
_____
_____
_____
_____
_____

Current weight _____

Would you like your weight to be different? _____ If yes, what? _____

Measurements of waist? _____ Hips? _____ Thigh? _____

Did you reach your goal? _____

What will this mean for you? _____

_____

_____

_____

_____

_____

_____

_____

_____

_____

_____

_____

_____

_____

_____

_____

_____

_____

_____

_____

_____

_____

_____

_____

_____

_____

_____

$\mathcal{R}$ E S O U R C E S

Clean up your diet by Max Tomlinson

www.heart.org American Heart Association website

Integrative Nutrition by Joshua Rosenthal

www.beststemcellnews.com Primordial Food by Dr. Christian Drapeau

"Pesticides in drinking water." National Pesticide Telecommunications Network. N.p., 01 July 2000

http://myplace.frontier.com/~felipe2/id18.html

Millionaire & Healthy; By Thomas J. Rundquist

http://www.motherjones.com/tom-philpott/2013/01/coca-cola-vitamin-water-obesity

www.nih.gov

www.DrWeil.com

www.mahopachealthcoaching.com

www.badmikeys.com

www.karenmayo.net

www.hemlockhillfarm.com

www.doctoroz.com

www.wholefoods.com

Made in the USA
Lexington, KY
14 November 2015